Clean Eating

Lose Weight with 172 Recipes That Are Delicious & Easy to Make (SMASH Food Cravings & Enjoy Eating Healthy)

by Olivia Rogers

Copyright © 2017 By Olivia Rogers
All rights reserved. No part of this book may be reproduced in any form without permission in writing from the author. No part of this publication may be reproduced or transmitted in any form or by any means, mechanic, electronic, photocopying, recording, by any storage or retrieval system, or transmitted by email without the permission in writing from the author and publisher.
For information regarding permissions write to author at
Olivia@TheMenuAtHome.com
Reviewers may quote brief passages in review.

Please note that credit for the images used in this book go to the respective owners. You can view this at: TheMenuAtHome.com/image-list

Olivia Rogers
TheMenuAtHome.com

Table of Contents

Who Is This Book For? — 11
What Will This Book Teach You? — 11
Introduction — 12
Chapter 1: No Sugar — 14
Chapter 2: No Refined Flour — 18
Chapter 3: No Trans Fats — 20
Chapter 4: No Fast Food — 22
Chapter 5: More Fiber — 23
Chapter 6: More Protein — 25
Chapter 7: More Healthy Fats — 27
Chapter 8: Meal Recipes — 30
1. Arugula Soup — 30
2. Thai Chicken and Mushroom Broth — 31
3. Sweet Cabbage Salad — 32
4. Sea Bass with Sizzled Ginger, Chili & Spring Onions — 33
5. Savory Beet Soup — 33
6. Sweet and Sour Chicken — 34
7. Vegetarian Stuffed Mushrooms — 35
8. Jam Biscuits — 36
9. Scallops in Parchment with Fennel, Tomatoes, and Olives — 37
10. Thai Prawn Curry — 38
11. Spicy Falafel — 39
12. Parmesan Spring Chicken — 40
13. Marinated Smoked Salmon with Poppy Seeds — 41
14. Garlic & Basil Ciabatta — 42

15. Tomato and Thyme Cod _____ 43
16. Pan-Fried Scallops with Lime & Coriander _____ 44
17. Creamed Spinach _____ 45
18. Scones with Clotted Cream and Jam _____ 46
19. Cheese, Leek and Potato Tortilla _____ 47
20. Couscous with Garlicky Grilled Tilapia _____ 48
21. Asparagus and Bulgur with Lemony Baked Salmon _____ 49
22. Barbecued Chipotle-Marinated Pork Sandwiches _____ 50
23. Pecorino & Ravioli with Arugula _____ 51
24. Chops au Poivre _____ 52
25. Balsamic Onion Quesadillas & Turkey _____ 53
26. Black Beans with Southwestern Salad _____ 54
27. Cornmeal-Crusted Chicken Nuggets with Blackberry Mustard _____ 55
28. Greek Salad with Sardines _____ 56
29. Troy's Hana-Style Sauce with Ginger-Steamed Fish _____ 57
30. Cube Steak with Mushroom-Sherry Sauce _____ 59
31. Marmalade Chicken _____ 60
32. Creamy Piccata Sauce with Poached Salmon _____ 61
33. Pepita-Lime Butter with Salmon _____ 62
34. Moo Shu Vegetables _____ 63
35. Cheddar Soup, Broccoli & Cannellini Bean _____ 64
36. Sweet Potato Hash with Chili-Glazed Pork _____ 65
37. Pan Salsa & Chili-Rubbed Steaks _____ 66
38. Japanese Chicken-Scallion Rice Bowl _____ 67
39. Fettuccine with Shiitake Mushrooms & Basil _____ 68
40. Rhubarb Chutney with Turkey Cutlets _____ 69

41. Maple-Chili Glazed Pork Medallions _____ 70
42. Black Bean-Salmon Stir-Fry _____ 71
43. Sun-Dried Tomato Wraps & Turkey and Corn _____ 72
44. Skillet Chicken with Apples & Cranberries _____ 73
45. Quick Pastrami Hash & Eggs _____ 74
46. Black Bean-Smothered Sweet Potatoes _____ 75
47. Port Sauce & Seared Steak with Pan-Roasted Grape _____ 76
48. Smoky Maple-Mustard Salmon _____ 78
49. Soba Noodles and Spicy Pork _____ 79
50. Black Bean Salad & Zesty Shrimp _____ 80
51. Sicilian Olive Chicken _____ 81
52. Seared Salmon with Green Peppercorn Sauce _____ 82
53. Crab Roll _____ 83
54. Green Beans with Pesto & Poached Cod _____ 84
55. Kale Salad with Preserved Lemon & Walnuts _____ 85
56. Olive Oil & Herb Mashed Potatoes _____ 86
57. Salmon Cakes with Olives, Lemon & Dill _____ 87
58. Three Sisters Succotash _____ 88
59. Turkey Kofta with Tahini Sauce _____ 89
60. Spiced Salmon with Chili Sauce _____ 90
61. Fish and Baby Tomato Bake _____ 91
62. Pork Kebabs with Chimichurri _____ 92
63. Sautéed Minute Steaks _____ 93
64. Beef Steak with Mushrooms _____ 94
65. Venetian Style Pasta _____ 95
66. Pork Panfry _____ 96
67. Sealed Hake with Olive Salsa _____ 97

68. Sweet and Sour Pork _____ 98
69. Broccoli and Cauliflower Primavera _____ 98
70. Bacon Wraps _____ 99
71. Beef and Broccoli Stir-Fry _____ 100
72. Roast Sea Bass with Orange and Honey _____ 101
73. Broiled Tilapia Parmesan _____ 102
74. Teriyaki Fried Rice with Chicken _____ 103
75. Spicy Beans and Rice _____ 104
76. Onion and Cheese Tarts _____ 104
77. Tomato Tartlets _____ 105
78. Curried Broccoli and Cabbage _____ 106
79. Mushroom and Cabbage Stroganoff _____ 107
80. Summer Cabbage Soup with Sausages _____ 108
81. North African Cabbage _____ 109
82. Cheese Crumpets _____ 109
83. Four Bean Salad _____ 110
84. Singed Steak, Tomato and Blue Cheese Salad _____ 111
85. Potato, Bacon and Avocado Salad _____ 112
86. Mexican Salad _____ 113
87. Garlic Chicken with Egg Plant Salad _____ 113
88. Cod Served with Corn, Beans and Pesto _____ 114
89. Walnut, Beets and Goat Cheese Salad _____ 115
90. Steak Salad with Mango Cubes _____ 116
91. Spinach and Garlic Vinaigrette _____ 117
92. Quinoa served with Mushrooms, Kale, and Sweet Potatoes 118
93. Pea Risotto with Baked Spinach _____ 118
94. Braised Chicken with Radish and Baby Carrots _____ 119

95. Pumpkin Soup _____ 120

96. Chickpeas with Roasted Tomatoes and Raisins _____ 121

97. Chicken and Noodle Soup _____ 122

98. Cumin Chicken on a Bed of Black Beans_____ 123

99. Meatball Soup with Escarole _____ 124

100. Chickpea Salad with Red Chili Flakes_____ 125

101. Sautéed Mushroom and Chicken Sandwiched in a Bran Bread _____ 126

102. Grilled Chicken Thighs on a Bed of Brown Rice _____ 127

103. Egg and Rocket Pizza _____ 127

104. Oats with Fruits and Nuts Topped with Greek Yogurt ____ 128

105. Thai Prawn Fried Rice_____ 129

106. Baked Sea Bass with Lemon and Capers _____ 130

107. Confetti Pesto Pasta with Diced Chicken and Green Beans _____ 131

108. Steak and Pepper Tacos _____ 132

109. Shrimp and Avocado Rice Bowl _____ 133

110. Lemon Walnut Chicken _____ 134

111. Spinach Mushroom Pizza _____ 135

112. Chickpea Tagine_____ 137

113. Penne with Broccoli and Ricotta _____ 138

114. Cumin Salmon with Yogurt-Cucumber Sauce _____ 139

115. Hearty Roast Beef Panini_____ 140

116. Turkey Meatloaf with Walnuts and Sage _____ 141

117. Slow Cooker Moroccan Chicken with Olives_____ 143

118. Chicken Piccata _____ 144

119. Slow Cooker African Chicken Stew _____ 145

120. Spicy Olive and Turkey Pita Sandwich _____ 146
121. Peppered Bacon Chickoli _____ 147
122. Slow Cooked Low Carb Mexi Chicken _____ 148
123. Slow Cooker Carnitas _____ 149
124. Beef and Vegetable Parmesan_____ 150
125. Slow Cooked Tilapia Parmesan _____ 151
126. Slow Cooker Thai Curry Beef _____ 151
127. Slow Cooked Stuffed Gammon _____ 152
128. Slow Cooker Breakfast Casserole _____ 153
129. Apple Cinnamon Slow Cooker Oatmeal_____ 154
130. Slow Cooker Sausage and Egg Breakfast Casserole____ 155
131. Savory Bean Cake _____ 156
132. Slow Cooked Fish Cakes _____ 157
133. Low Carb Slow Cooker Jambalaya _____ 158
134. Low Carb Crock Pot Chili _____ 159
135. Cheesy Cauliflower Soup _____ 160
136. Winter Vegetable Soup _____ 161
137. Serene Day Beef Soup_____ 162
138. Creamy Chicken and Peppers Enchilada _____ 163
139. Slow Cooked Tamale Bake_____ 163
140. Cabbage Roll Stew_____ 164
141. Slow Cooker Boston Baked Beans _____ 165
142. Spinach, artichoke and Kale Dip_____ 166
143. Sweet Potato Breakfast Casserole_____ 167
144. Wheat-Free Frittata _____ 168
145. Pancakes_____ 169
146. Oatmeal Banana Bake _____ 170

147. Biscuits _____ 171
148. Biscuit Gravy _____ 172
149. Cauliflower Pizza Crust _____ 172
150. Flat Bread _____ 173
151. Enchilada Casserole _____ 174
152. Chicken and Dumplings _____ 175
153. Chicken Strips _____ 175
154. Quinoa Casserole _____ 176
155. Flaxseed Wraps _____ 177
156. Macaroni and Cheese _____ 178
157. Meatloaf _____ 179
158. Cauliflower Mashed Potatoes _____ 179
159. Crusty Chicken Casserole _____ 180
160. Cheese Crackers _____ 181
161. Pretzels _____ 182
162. Thai Salmon Soup _____ 182
163. Tomato Soup _____ 183
164. Coconut Crusted Salmon _____ 184
165. Peanut Crusted Chicken _____ 185
166. Cheeseburger Pie _____ 186
167. Broccoli Cheese Soup _____ 187
168. Chicken Broccoli Casserole _____ 188
169. Cheesecake _____ 189
170. Peanut Squares _____ 190
171. Chocolate Cupcakes _____ 191
172. Blueberry Coffee Cake _____ 192
Conclusion _____ 193

Final Words _____ *193*
Disclaimer _____ *195*

Who Is This Book For?

This book suits everyone, from the skilled, gourmet low-cal cook out to stretch their culinary ambitions, to the novice skimming for ideal low-calorie fare. You've got it all from an expert! If you are planning to switch to a low-calorie healthy lifestyle then you probably cannot win without the help of this compelling cookbook! Those of you who have been planning to switch to a healthy lifestyle can benefit immensely from this book.

The low-cal recipes we have compiled are a pleasant change from the dull and boring diet food that you have been eating. This is indeed a tasty way to lose weight. A complete guide for people who are looking to cut their weight without having to go through much of a diet plan, this book contains a list of a wide variety of recipes. This text is an absolute treat for those who are not big fans of standing in the kitchen for long hours in the hope of satisfying their hunger.

Moreover, people who like to read facts about what they eat and want to be aware of what nutrients are present in their diet can also benefit from this book and increase their knowledge about different ingredients which are used for preparing various recipes. Some recipes in this book have been listed for those readers as well who like to put their food in the oven for a few hours and wait while it cooks slowly. Those of you who would like to know more about dressing their food and garnishing it with vegetables and salads can also learn a lot from this text. All in all, this text is a complete guide for different groups of people, who want to shed their weight without having to sacrifice their appetite.

What Will This Book Teach You?

Not only will you enjoy **Couscous with Garlicky Grilled Tilapia**, but you'll also sift through some of the best food, chapter after another, finding mouthwatering meals like **Arugula Soup, Black Bean-Salmon Stir-Fry, Skillet Chicken with Apples & Cranberries** and **Three Sisters Succotash**. The recipes in this book, many of which can be prepared for one and less than 20 minutes, are super simple and are geared towards satisfying your relentless appetite for overly high calorie meals without blowing your waistline. The biggest message we want to give out is being healthy need not mean giving up on the good things in life. We don't think healthy = non-palatable, bland food. Our intent is to spice up your diet in a way that you eat a tasty meal which will titillate your taste buds, yet not add to your weight.

This book brings to you some easy to cook low-cal recipes that will help you lose weight without punishing your taste buds. This book is all about preparing health friendly recipes and enjoying them. Going through the next few pages will teach you how you can make delicious low-fat dishes without going through much difficulty. The main ingredients of each of the recipe have been listed before the procedure and the exact quantities of all the contents have also been displayed.

At the end of each recipe, a fun fact about an ingredient or the recipe has also been giving to make your journey through this book more joyous and less boring. Most of the recipes which have been discussed are quick to prepare, however, a couple of slow cook foods have also been listed for the lovers of such recipes. The dishes which have been discussed here can be used for dinners as well as lunch and some can even be served for brunch. The recipes are from cultures all around the world and hence, will be very appealing for the readers, and that's a fact.

Introduction

When your stomach begins grumbling and the cravings set in, you know it's time to find the healthy yet low calorie foods that make each bite count. This cookbook is packed with incredibly tasty, low-calorie recipes that the entire family will love. It offers you an unparalleled variety of meals and tips to eat healthfully—for a lifetime! Also, the recipes in this book clock in at less than 300 calories. Most of all they are impressively easy to make and take the guesswork out of calorie counting and portion control. You already know it doesn't get better than this—to get a cookbook that brings you complete low calorie recipes that maintain a balanced eating approach—naturally!

The biggest challenge that man faces in terms of threats to his existence is adverse health conditions. Cosseted by technology and comforted by the materialistic supports, we have evolved into a race that is perennially engaged in the chase of that perfect life. We grapple around us to amass wealth and other superficial possessions, but we tend to conveniently forget and ignore that old proverb that we had learnt while in school, that our biggest wealth is indeed good health. This especially holds true for people stuck in conventional jobs that demand them to slave upwards of 12 hours a day, perched in front of computer screens. Needless to say, putting in quality time for some good old physical exercise is out of the question. An even more alarming trend is the change in nutritional pattern that has accompanied this fast paced, harebrained style of working.

It will be redundant to even imagine that people can consume food that is actually good for them; they simply cannot find the time to do so. Eventually what happens is that they gorge on fast food and aerated soft drinks that are nothing but glorified empty calories packaged in mighty sounding marketing drivel promising you the best of nature! Couldn't muster the time or energy to prepare a proper meal, grab a quick burger. Did not find the gap to have a juice? Get a soft drink. Need to stay up overnight for work? No problem, get one of those hyper energy drinks that get you high! This is the mindset that has plagued our generation, and if measures are not taken to curb this slip, be sure that it will spell doom for our race. But for those of you, who are genuinely concerned about your health, fear not, for now you have this book. This book is a collection of fabulous low-calorie recipes that you can whip in less than 20 minutes. These are designed for those individuals who are perpetually caught in the fast lane. And what's more, this is not simply a list of recipes after monotonous recipe of greens! Far from it, this is a compilation of dishes that are a gastronomic delight. And to top it all off, we have also included little tips and fun facts for each recipe that is bound to entice you.

The main purpose of the recipes in this book is weight loss. The recipes tackle weight loss through their low-calorie levels which is a sure way of losing weight. Contrary to popular belief that low-calorie foods are bland, the recipes in this book produce dishes which are tasty, nutritious and healthy. Most ingredients included have several other health benefits which are an addition to losing weight. The beauty of these recipes is that, you do not need hours preparing the food, all you need is twenty minutes; or less. If you want to lose weight but you cannot resist food, this book is just for you. If you are looking for a number of low-fat recipes which are rich in nutrients as well as quite easy to cook, you have come to the right place. Most of the low-calorie recipes are prepared by using low-fat ingredients including dry fruits, fresh vegetables, low-sodium milk, lean meat and fish. Vegetables have been used in most cases to dress the dishes and add to the nutritional value.

The main reason for the accumulation of fat in human body is the consumption of high calorie diet which is rich in carbs. Sugar containing foods, creams and desserts are rich in such dangerous elements and therefore, result in weight gain. The recipes which are discussed in the following chapters do not contain any of these contents, but have the necessary proteins and vitamins which are required to make a human body work. Combining such harmless ingredients with contents like yogurt, almonds, walnuts and lime juice helps in keeping the fat at bay and digesting the food more efficiently. Moreover, garlic, onions, avocado and jalapenos have also been found to be very good for the functioning of heart and maintaining the density of the blood so the dishes discussed in this book are perfect for people of all ages. If you've been trying diet after diet to lose weight, only to have those extra pounds stay stubbornly in place, it's time to try a new approach.

The truth is that there's no secret diet that's going to burn away fat. What you need to do is make a few changes to the way you eat and make those changes a long-term habit. That is, you have to nourish your body and feed it what it really needs in order to lose weight. Instead of suffering through strict diets, you should eat as much as you want—just make sure what you are eating is healthy. In this book, you'll also learn the 7 key changes that will *guarantee* weight loss. In addition to learning about the changes you need to make, you'll get easy recipes to help make the transition easier. So, read on and learn how you can make those pounds melt away once and for all! I also hope to teach you some amazing slow cooking recipes that you can do in your crock-pot, if you wish! The best part is that they are all low-carb, so they aren't going to break your current diet and weight loss plans! Do you need a *strong* kick-start with your weight loss? Are you ready for a full body transformation? Do you just wish that your fat would just fall off *effortlessly?* If you answered "Yes" to any of those questions – **this book is for you!**

I am going to share with you some of the best recipes that are going to HELP you with your weight loss. In these recipes, you may see some ingredients that are new to you. We use almond flour as a great alternative to wheat flour. Any nut flour will work including almond, hazelnut, or walnut. Just grind the nuts to fine flour in your food processor. We use stevia as a sweetener and coconut oil because they are healthy alternatives. We have included breakfast ideas and snack, old favorites and something new. All are easy to prepare. With these recipes, it is easy to eat wheat-free from morning until night. During your time invested in reading this book, you will come across scrumptious, low calorie recipes that will do two things for you; satisfy your taste buds AND help you lose weight. Follow your heart, and enjoy food! So, what are you waiting for? Roll up your chef's sleeves and get down to it! Bon Appetite! Written by Olivia Rogers, a well-respected cookbook author, this book contains incredibly nutritious and satisfying low calorie recipes, carefully chosen by to help you drop those extra pounds and boost your metabolism. Admittedly, there are millions of low calorie cookbooks in the market today and as you wade through this myriad; you want to keep a great low-calorie book at the top of your list. Ready? Let's move!

Chapter 1: No Sugar

If you had to pick just one weight loss technique, get rid of sugar. White sugar is the biggest cause of weight gain in most people. This is not to say it is the *only* cause but it is at the top of the list. Just by cutting out sugar, you can actually help your body to burn more calories per day. In one recent study, participants were divided into groups. Each group at the same total number of calories and did the same intensity of exercise. The difference? How much sugar and refined flours they ate. Those who ate low sugar/refined flour diets (i.e.- sugar and refined flour made up less than 10% of total calories) were burning an average of 365 more calories per day than those who ate more sugar and refined flour. That means that right now, this very day, you can burn more than 300 extra calories per day just by *not* eating sugar!

This doesn't mean you have to give up all sweet things. You can enjoy fruits and many healthy sugar substitutes. The main thing you need to avoid is *added* sugar. That means if sugar is an ingredient in the food you are eating, don't eat that food or make your own version of it using healthier alternatives to sugar. Here are 2 sugar free recipes to help you give up sugar without giving up your favorite treats:

Grape Soda

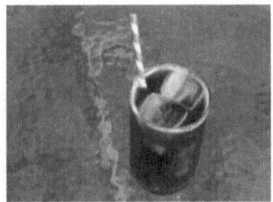

- ¾ lb. Seedless Black Grapes
- ¼ lb. Blueberries
- ½ cup Water
- Juice from ½ Lemon
- Sparkling Water

Directions

1. In a pot over medium-high heat, stir together first 4 ingredients. Let simmer 20 minutes, smashing fruit as they cook. Pour mixture into a food processor. Pulse until pureed. Refrigerate mixture until chilled. To serve, mix equal parts fruit mixture and sparkling water.

Pop Tarts

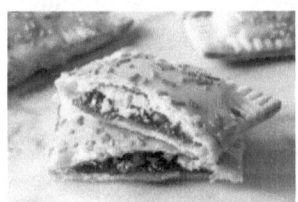

- 1 ½ cups Almond Meal
- ¼ cup Oat Flour
- 2 Tbsps. Butter

- ¼ tsp Baking Soda
- ¼ tsp Salt
- 1 tsp Vanilla Extract
- 1 Egg (beaten)
- 1 cup Raspberries
- 1 Tbsp. Lemon Juice
- 2 Tbsps. Unsweetened Apple Sauce
- 2 Tbsps. (+ 1 tsp) Molasses
- 1/16 tsp Unflavored Gelatin

Directions

1. Preheat oven to 350°F. Combine baking soda, salt, almond and oat flour in a bowl. Cut in cold butter in chunks. Mix with a fork (or your hands) until mixture is clumpy. In a separate bowl, whisk egg until frothy. Slowly drizzle into flour mixture, stirring to combine. Make sure dough remains crumbly (you may not need all the egg). Press dough into a ball. Chill in refrigerator 30 minutes.

2. In a blender, puree lemon juice, applesauce, vanilla extract, raspberries, gelatin, molasses and a dash of salt. Once pureed, pour into a microwave-safe cup. Microwave 4 minutes. Let cool. Whisk puree until evenly blended. Divide dough into 3-4 even balls. Place each ball between 2 pieces of parchment paper. Roll out into thin squares. Remove the top piece of parchment paper. Use a pizza cutter to cut pop tart sized rectangles out of the dough.

3. Arrange rectangles on a parchment paper lined baking sheet. Brush rectangles with remaining egg mixture. Divide raspberry puree evenly amongst half of the rectangles. Spread puree evenly. Leave about ½" space around the edges. Place the rectangles without raspberry on top of the raspberry filled rectangles. Press edges down with your fingers to seal. Poke holes all over the top. Bake 20 minutes for pop tarts that will be eaten immediately. Bake 15 minutes for pop tarts that will be toasted and eaten later.

Read This FIRST - 100% FREE BONUS

FOR A LIMITED TIME ONLY – Get Olivia's best-selling book *"The #1 Cookbook: Over 170+ of the Most Popular Recipes Across 7 Different Cuisines!"* absolutely FREE!

Readers have absolutely loved this book because of the wide variety of recipes. It is highly recommended you check these recipes out and see what you can add to your home menu!

Once again, as a big thank-you for downloading this book, I'd like to offer it to you *100% FREE for a LIMITED TIME ONLY!*

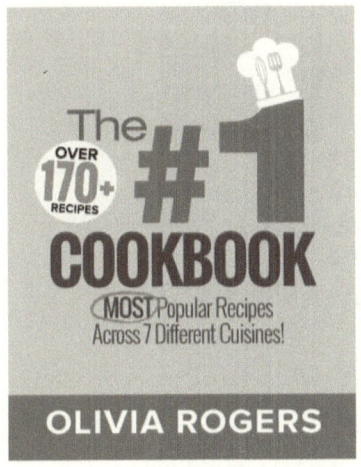

Get your free copy at:

TheMenuAtHome.com/Bonus

Chapter 2: No Refined Flour

Refined flour is the second biggest enemy to weight loss. In the same study mentioned in the first chapter, those who saw the greatest improvement to fat burning were the ones who cut out sugar *and* refined flours. Refined flour is the main ingredient in most processed breads and pastries. It's the key ingredient in white bread, cookies, cakes, pizzas, and all the other junk food you shouldn't be eating but find it hard to resist. But by resisting those refined flour foods (in addition to cutting out sugar), you can burn even more fat each day.

I won't lie. At first, you will miss it (especially sugar). But after 2 weeks or so, you are going to start appreciating the taste of nutritious whole grains and naturally sweet foods. Eventually, you enjoy those healthier flavors more than the refined sugar and flour you were eating before. To ease the transition, here are 2 recipes for 2 of your favorite refined flour foods:

White Bread

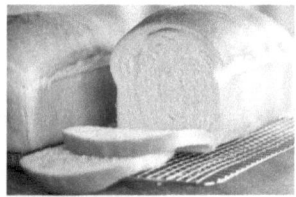

- 3 ½ cups White Whole Grain Flour
- 1/3 cup Vital Wheat Gluten
- 4 tsp Instant Yeast
- 2 ½ cups Warm Water (120°F)
- 1 Tbsp. Salt
- 1/3 cup Olive Oil
- 1/3 cup Mashed Banana
- 4 tsp Lemon Juice
- 2 ½ cups White Whole Grain Flour

Directions

1. Blend together first 3 ingredients. Add water and mix until dough comes together. Cover and let rest 10 minutes. In a bowl, whisk together oil, banana, lemon juice and salt for 1 minute. Beat into dough mixture. Add remaining flour 1 cup at a time, beating to combine.

2. Knead dough 10-15 minutes until smooth and even ball forms. Divide into 2 even pieces. Place in 2 greased loaf pans, pressing to push dough into corners. Cover and let rise in a warm place until doubled in size (about 40 minutes). Preheat oven to 350°F. Bake 30 minutes.

Mac 'n' Cheese

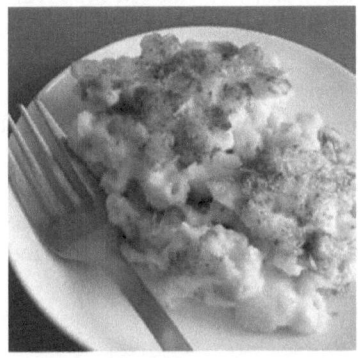

- 2 cups Whole Grain Macaroni (or other pasta)
- 2 Tbsps. Whole Grain Flour
- 1/8 tsp Pepper
- 1 ½ cups Whole Milk
- 1 cup Grated Mozzarella
- 1 cup Grated Smoked Cheddar
- 1 large Carrot (sliced)
- 1 Zucchini (diced)
- 1 Onion (diced)
- 1 Garlic Clove (minced)
- Olive Oil

Directions

1. Heat 2 tablespoons oil in a large pot over medium-high heat. Add onion. Cook 2 minutes, stirring occasionally. Add carrot. Cook 6 minutes, stirring occasionally. Add zucchini. Cook 3 minutes, stirring occasionally. In a separate pot, boil water and cook pasta.

2. Add 3 tablespoons oil, flour, garlic and pepper to veggies. Cook 2 minutes, stirring constantly. Stir in milk. Add cheese a handful at a time, stirring constantly to combine. Reduce heat to a simmer. Cover and let simmer until thickened (about 5-8 minutes). Drain pasta and stir into cheese sauce. Serve.

Chapter 3: No Trans Fats

The third enemy on the list is Trans-fat. Unlike saturated and unsaturated fats, Trans-fat has been chemically altered during processing. This chemical change turns it into something that your body can't handle. Rather than get rid of it, though, your body chooses to just store it as fat. Trans-fat is the one fat that does actually make you fat. Saturated fats (in moderation) and unsaturated fats have both been shown to help you *lose* weight.

So, the bad news is: no more trans-fat foods. But the good news is: you can enjoy unsaturated fats to satisfy your cravings for fatty foods. Trans fats are typically found in pre-prepared fried chicken, donuts, and other fried foods. It's also found margarine and other "buttery" foods that don't actually use butter. Always check labels to make sure there are *zero* Trans fats and try out these 2 recipes below for a healthier alternative to fried chicken and donuts:

Fried Chicken

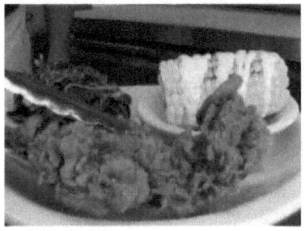

- 1 ½ cup Whole Grain Flour
- 1 tsp Ground Ginger
- ½ tsp Paprika
- ½ tsp Cinnamon
- ½ tsp Nutmeg
- ½ tsp Salt
- 2 Skinless Bone-In Chicken Breasts
- 2 Skinless Bone-In Chicken Thighs
- 2 Skinless Chicken Drumsticks
- ¼ cup Olive Oil

Directions

1. Add first 6 ingredients to a re-sealable bag. Close and shake to mix. Sprinkle salt evenly over each piece of chicken. Add chicken to bag one piece at a time. Seal and shake to coat. Remove chicken and pat off excess flour. Repeat with each piece.

2. Place coated chicken in a baking dish. Cover. Chill 2 hours. Let stand at room temperature 30 minutes. Put chicken in flour mixture bag 1 piece at a time. Shake to coat. Pat off excess flour.

3. Heat oil in a large pan over medium-high heat. Add chicken to pan. Reduce heat to medium-low. Cook 25 minutes. Turn every 5 minutes. Drain chicken on paper towels for 5 minutes. (Note: oil can be reserved for future use with this same recipe).

Donuts

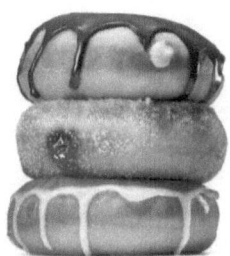

- 3 Eggs
- 3 Tbsps. Almond Oil (+ more for greasing)
- 2 Tbsps. Maple Syrup
- 1 ripe Banana
- ½ tsp Vanilla Extract
- 1 cup Almond Flour
- ¼ cup Quinoa Flour
- ¼ tsp Salt
- ½ tsp Cinnamon
- ¼ tsp Baking Soda
- ½ tsp Nutmeg
- 1/3 cup Dark Chocolate Chips
- 1 Tbsp. Coconut Oil
- ¼ cup Cocoa Powder
- Shredded Coconut & Sliced Almonds (optional)

Directions

1. Preheat oven to 350°F. Grease a donut pan liberally with almond oil and set aside. In a blender, pulse together wet ingredients (except coconut oil) until smooth. Add dry ingredients (except cocoa powder and chocolate chips). Pulse until smooth. Let rest 10 minutes.

2. Fill donut molds 2/3 of the way with batter. Bake 5 minutes. Remove. Brush with almond oil. Return to oven. Bake 5-6 more minutes (or until inserted toothpick comes out clean). Remove donuts from mold, let cool.

3. Melt together chocolate chips and coconut oil in a double boiler. Whisk in cocoa powder. Use tongs to dip donuts into chocolate glaze until completely coated. Let extra drip off. Roll donuts in coconut flakes and sliced almonds. Arrange on a platter. Let cool.

Chapter 4: No Fast Food

Not all fast food is bad for you. There are some restaurant chains that take pride in using real, natural ingredients in their meals. But, in general, fast food restaurants use all 3 ingredients we talked about in the first 3 chapters. It's a triple-attack of all these enemies to weight loss. Plus, it doesn't taste half as good as the versions you can make at home using real, fresh ingredients.

If you're really craving some quick take out, check the restaurant's website for nutrition information to see what ingredients they use. Check for meals that have no Trans fats, no sugar, and no refined flour. That's going to be hard (or impossible) to find for most fast food restaurants. But there are a few good restaurants out there if you do your research. Otherwise, just satisfy your fast food cravings at home by trying out the 2 recipes below for a classic burger & fries' dinner:

Cheeseburger

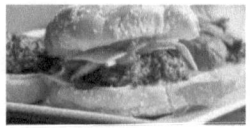

- 1 lb. Ground Lamb (or Turkey)
- ¼ lb. Quinoa (cooked)
- ¼ tsp Garlic Powder
- ½ tsp Onion Powder
- 1 Tbsp. Worcestershire Sauce
- 2 Tbsps. Dijon Mustard
- ½ tsp Pepper
- 4 slices Smoked Cheddar
- Whole Grain Buns (grilled)
- 1 cup large Spinach Leaves

Directions

1. In a large bowl, mix together all ingredients by hand. Divide and form into 4 patties. Don't press them too tightly. Just shape lightly until formed. Prepare a grill for medium-high heat. Grill patties 2-3 minutes per side (or until cooked to your liking).

2. After flipping patty, place a slice of cheddar on each one. Place buns on grill (cut-side down). Grill buns 1-2 minutes. Remove buns. Arrange a layer of spinach on each bottom slice. Place burger patty on top of spinach. Cover with top of bun. Add any additional condiments or veggies as desired.

Curly Fries

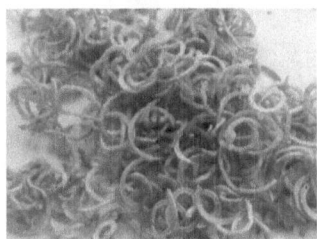

- Turnips (peeled)
- Egg
- Olive Oil
- Garlic Powder
- Paprika

Directions

1. Preheat oven to 400°F. Use a spiralizer to cut turnips into curls. Whisk together equal parts egg and olive oil. Season with garlic powder and paprika to taste. Toss turnip curls in oil mixture. Arrange on a baking sheet. Roast in oven 20 minutes. Flip 2-3 times while roasting.

Chapter 5: More Fiber

Losing weight isn't just about cutting food out of your diet. It's equally important to make sure you are replacing those foods with healthier alternatives. The good news is you can really eat as much as you want. Don't worry about counting calories. Focus instead on counting nutrients. Make sure you are getting enough fiber, protein, and unsaturated fats from a variety of fresh, natural sources. Fiber is an essential tool to help your body lose weight. It helps you burn fat in a few different ways. First of all, it improves digestion so that you digest food more efficiently. It also helps fight cravings. This is because fiber digests more slowly than sugar, Trans fats, or refined flour. Because it spends more time digesting, you feel full longer (meaning less cravings and between-meal snacking).

For the same reason, it also helps stabilize your blood sugar levels. Rather than sending a burst of energy to your body (like sugar does), it sends a steady, stable stream of energy. This means you won't experience the spikes and crashes in energy levels that you do with sugary foods. These crashes in energy levels are one of the leading causes of cravings. Your body panics and starts craving sugary foods just to get energy levels back up. By eating more fiber, you avoid these crashes (and the cravings that come with them). You should be eating 25-30 grams of fiber per day. Try out these 2 recipes to get more fiber in your diet:

Chocolate Cake

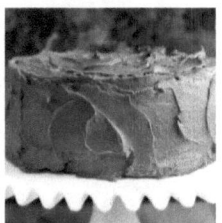

- 1 cup Quinoa (cooked)
- 1 cup Oat Flour
- 1/3 cup Milk
- 4 large Eggs
- 1 tsp Vanilla
- ¾ cup Butter (melted)
- 1 cup Mashed Banana
- ½ cup Unsweetened Applesauce
- 1 cup Cocoa Powder
- 1 ½ tsp Baking Powder
- ½ tsp Baking Soda
- ½ tsp Salt

Directions

1. Preheat oven to 350°F. Grease 2 cake dishes (8") and line with parchment paper. In a blender, pulse together eggs, milk, and vanilla.

Add melted butter, banana, applesauce, and cooked quinoa. Blend until smooth.

2. In a bowl, whisk together cocoa, baking powder, baking soda, and salt. Pour into blender and pulse until smooth. Divide batter evenly between the two greased dishes. Bake 40 minutes (or until inserted toothpick comes out clean).

"All-9" Smoothie

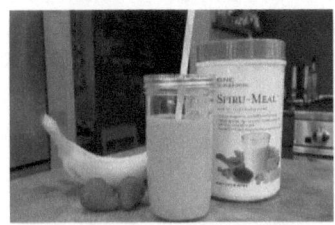

- 1 Avocado
- 1 cup Spinach
- ½ cup Chard
- ½ cup Kale
- ½ cup Carrots (chopped)
- 1 cup Strawberries
- 1 ripe Banana
- 1 Orange
- ½ cup Coconut Milk
- ½ cup Plain Greek Yogurt
- 2 tsp Vanilla Extract

Directions

1. Combine all ingredients together in a blender until smooth. Replace Greek yogurt with coconut milk for a more drinkable smoothie. Replace coconut milk with Greek yogurt for a thicker meal-replacement smoothie. Replace kale with spinach if the texture is too grainy for you.

Chapter 6: More Protein

Eating more protein is another great way to help you lose weight. Protein is an essential ingredient to building muscles. How does this relate to weight loss, you ask? Well, studies have shown that muscles burn more calories than fat. This means that the more muscles you have, the more calories you are burning (even when you aren't doing anything). Without protein, your body can't build muscle. But this isn't the only way protein helps you burn fat. It also fights cravings. Out of the 3 macronutrients—protein, fiber, and unsaturated fats—protein takes the longest to digest. This means it provides a long term, highly stable stream of energy.

So, you will feel full for hours after eating a high protein meal. You will also maintain a steady energy level which (as you learned in chapter 4) will help you fight off cravings for sugary foods. You should eat a minimum of about 60 grams of protein per day but you can eat as much as 1 gram per pound of body weight (if you are working out regularly). Try out the 2 protein-packed recipes below for a delicious and healthy way to eat more protein:

Fish Sticks

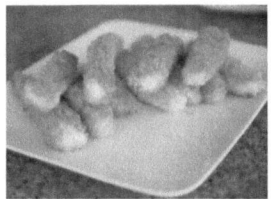

- 1 (18oz.) Skinless Salmon Fillet
- ½ cup Whole Grain Flour
- ½ tsp Salt
- ¼ tsp Black Pepper
- 3 Eggs
- 1 cup Grated Parmesan
- 1 cup Seasoned Whole Grain Bread Crumbs
- Olive Oil

Directions

1. Preheat oven to 450°F. Slice fillet in half. Slice each half into ½" strips. In a medium bowl, mix together flour, salt and pepper. In another bowl, beat eggs until frothy. In a third bowl, mix together bread crumbs and parmesan. Pour a 1/8" layer of oil into a baking dish.

2. Dip salmon strips into flour mixture. Pat to remove extra flour. Dip floured strip into egg. Then press into breadcrumbs until evenly coated. Arrange strips in baking dish. Turn to coat in oil. Bake 15-20 minutes. Serve with yogurt dressing.

Mixed Bean Burritos

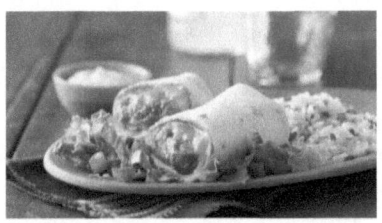

- ½ lb. canned White Beans (drained)
- ½ lb. canned Black Beans (drained)
- 1 cup Quinoa (cooked)
- 3 Garlic Cloves (minced, divided)
- 1 Tomato (diced)
- 1 Onion (diced)
- 1 cup Fresh Spinach (chopped)
- 1 tsp Cumin Powder
- 1 tsp Crushed Red Pepper Flakes
- 1 Avocado (peeled, diced)
- ½ tsp chili powder
- Olive Oil
- Salt to taste
- Sour Cream to serve
- 4 large Whole Grain Tortillas

Directions

1. Heat a little oil in a pan over medium-high heat. Add onions. Cook 6 minutes, stirring often. Add 2 garlic cloves, tomato, chili powder and cumin. Cook 2 minutes, stirring constantly. Add beans and quinoa. Cook until warm. Remove from heat. Set aside.

2. In a small bowl, mash avocado with remaining garlic, red pepper flakes, and salt. Warm tortillas over a gas stove top or in microwave until warm. Divide bean mixture evenly among tortillas. Sprinkle in spinach. Spoon in guacamole. Add a dollop of sour cream. Fold. Serve.

Chapter 7: More Healthy Fats

For decades, we have been told that we have to cut out fat if we want to lose fat. Unfortunately, this has led to countless "healthy" low-fat versions of foods. In order to make up for the missing flavor in low fat foods, manufacturers usually add sugar. As you learned in the first chapter, sugar is the leading cause of weight gain for most people. So, by replacing healthy fats with sugar, manufacturers are actually creating a *more* fattening food than the original.

Always buy the full fat versions of food (unless it contains Trans fats). You should eat about 15-20 grams of fat per day. The majority of this (about 90%) should come from unsaturated fats. The rest should come from saturated fat. Healthy fats keep you feeling full and help slow the rate at which you absorb energy. This helps stabilize your energy levels (which you now know helps fight cravings).

This means it is best to pair fats with your naturally sweet foods. Eat fruits mixed with ingredients high in unsaturated fats in order to slow the rate at which you use up the fruit sugars. This will help keep you energized throughout the day. Foods rich in healthy fats are also the best way to fight off cravings for unhealthy fatty foods. For example: eat a bowl of guacamole instead of French fries. Try out the 2 recipes below for some tasty ways to add more healthy fats to your diet.

Coconut Shrimp Pasta

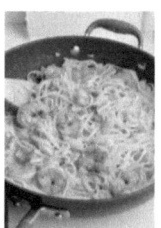

- 1 Tbsp. Olive Oil
- 1 Onion (thinly sliced)
- 1 large Bell Pepper (thinly sliced)
- 3 Garlic Cloves (thinly sliced)
- ½ cup White Wine
- 1 Tbsp. Balsamic Vinegar
- 1 (14oz.) can Coconut Milk
- 2 cups Broccoli (lightly steamed)
- 1 ¼ lbs. Shrimp (cooked, peeled)
- 4 cups Whole Grain Pasta (cooked)
- ½ cup Fresh Cilantro (chopped)
- 2 Tbsps. Sesame Seeds
- Salt & Pepper to taste

Directions

1. Heat oil in a large pan over medium-high heat. Add onion and bell pepper. Cook 6 minutes, stirring often. Add garlic. Cook 2 minutes, stirring constantly. Stir in vinegar and white wine. Cook until simmering. Simmer 2 minutes.

2. Stir in coconut milk. Bring to a boil. Reduce heat and simmer 10 minutes. Salt and pepper to taste. Stir in shrimp and broccoli. Cook 1 minute. Divide pasta among plates. Top with coconut shrimp. Drizzle extra sauce over. Sprinkle with cilantro and sesame seeds. Serve.

Granola Bars

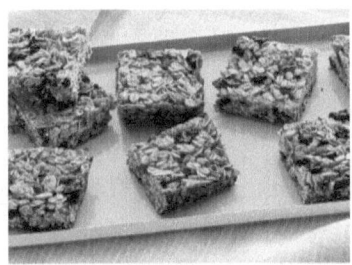

- 1 ½ cups Unsalted Roasted Almonds
- 1 Tbsp. Maple Syrup
- 1 Tbsp. Mashed Banana
- 3 Tbsps. Unsweetened Apple Sauce
- 1 tsp Vanilla Extract
- 1 cup Rolled Oats
- ½ cup Unsweetened Coconut Flakes
- ¼ cup Dried Cherries
- ¼ cup Dark Chocolate Chunks
- ¼ cup Sliced Almonds

Directions

1. In a food processor, pulse roasted almonds until smooth and buttery. Pour almond butter into a pot over medium heat with next 4 ingredients. Stir to combine. Remove from heat.

2. In a bowl, mix together remaining ingredients. Scrape almond mixture in and stir to combine. Spread mixture into an even 2"-3" layer in a baking dish. Let chill 2 hours. Cut into bars.

Chapter 8: Meal Recipes

1. Arugula Soup

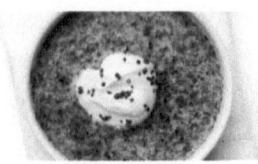

Arugula is a rich source of anti-oxidants and the best thing about the arugula soup is it is delicious, whether cold or hot!

Ingredients

- 1 (5-ounce) container baby arugula
- ½ medium onion, finely chopped
- ½ tablespoon olive oil
- 1 garlic clove, finely chopped
- 3 cups chicken broth (low sodium)
- ½ teaspoon cornstarch
- ¼ cup low-fat milk, evaporated
- 2 tablespoons plain Greek yogurt
- 1/8 cup mixed herbs, finely chopped
- 1 tablespoon chives, thinly sliced

Method

1. Heat the olive oil in a large saucepan over a medium- low heat. Add the chopped onion and garlic to the saucepan and cook for around five minutes till the onions turn translucent.

2. Next stir in the cornstarch followed by the chicken broth. Pour the evaporated milk into the saucepan next and mix all the ingredients well. Allow the mixture to simmer. Add the baby arugula followed by the chopped mixed herbs. Keep stirring till the leaves get wilted. Remove the saucepan from the heat at this point.

3. Using a lid, cover the saucepan and let the mixture rest for around five minutes. With the help of an immersion blender, blend the mixture until it reaches a smooth consistency. Transfer the soup to the serving bowls. Garnish each bowl with two teaspoons of Greek yogurt and the sliced chives and serve.

Tips/Notes

Arugula is packed with fiber, Vitamin C, vitamin A and vitamin K and is also an important source of potassium. It reduces the risk of heart diseases and cancer. Since Arugula is a source of vitamin K, it helps in the prevention of osteoporosis.

2. Thai Chicken and Mushroom Broth

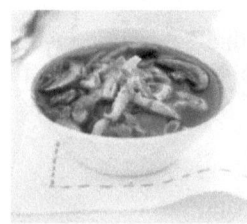

This refreshing broth is one of the best ways to recoup your immunity when you are down with the flu.

Ingredients

- 200 g cooked chicken, finely shredded
- 1-liter chicken stock
- 100 g Portobello mushrooms, thinly sliced
- 1 tablespoon Thai fish sauce
- 2 teaspoons sugar
- 1 tablespoon Thai red curry paste
- zest from 2 limes
- Juice from 2 limes
- A bunch of spring onions, thinly sliced
- Handful of fresh parsley, finely chopped

Method

1. Take a large saucepan and pour in the chicken stock, fish sauce, curry paste, lime juice, sugar and three fourths of the zest and mix them well. Bring the mixture to a boil.

2. Add the sliced mushrooms and spring onions to the boiling soup next. Let the soup simmer for around two minutes. Transfer the soup to the serving bowls. Garnish the soup with the remaining zest and the chopped parsley. Serve hot.

3. Sweet Cabbage Salad

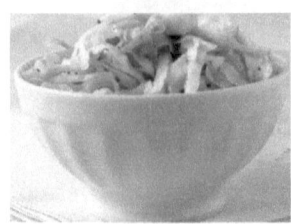

This is a healthier version of the Coleslaw sans the high fat content. This could be a light evening snack or be the crispy side dish for a heavy barbecue lunch.

Ingredients

- 3 cups shredded cabbage
- ½ cup chopped green bell pepper
- ½ cup shredded carrot
- ¼ cup chopped red onion
- ¼ cup white wine vinegar
- ¼ cup sugar
- 1 tablespoon olive oil
- ¼ teaspoon celery seeds
- ½ teaspoon dry mustard
- ¼ teaspoon salt

Method

1. Take a large bowl and add the cabbage, carrot, bell pepper and the onion to it and mix all the ingredients well. Take a small bowl. Add the sugar, olive oil, white wine vinegar, celery seeds, salt and dry mustard to it and mix them well.

2. Pour the dressing over the vegetables mixture and mix it in such a fashion that the dressing coats the salad evenly. Let it rest for some time before serving it.

Tips/Notes

Cabbage is full of vitamin K, which aids the functions of the brain and improves concentration power. Regular intake of cabbage prevents nerve damage and reduces the risk of Alzheimer's disease and dementia. The high potassium content in cabbage helps in regulating the blood pressure as well.

4. Sea Bass with Sizzled Ginger, Chili & Spring Onions

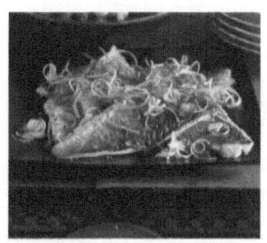

Being an excellent source of omega-3 fatty acids, this sizzling dish can help you battle against hypertension and high levels of blood cholesterol.

Ingredients

- 3 sea bass fillets, scaled
- A knob of ginger, peeled and thinly shredded
- 1 ½ tablespoons sunflower oil
- ½ tablespoon soy sauce
- 1 ½ garlic cloves, sliced thinly
- A bunch of spring onions, thinly shredded
- 1 ½ red chilies, deseeded and shredded thinly
- Salt and pepper, to taste

Method

1. Season the fillets well with salt and pepper and keep it aside. Heat ½ tablespoon sunflower oil in a frying pan. Fry the fillets in the oil for around five minutes till the skin turns golden brown. Flip it and cook it for another minute and transfer them to the serving plates.

2. Pour the remaining oil into the pan and fry the garlic, ginger and chilies for around two minutes till they turn golden. Remove the pan from the heat and add the shredded spring onions. Pour the contents of the frying pan over the fillets and drizzle with soy sauce. Serve hot.

5. Savory Beet Soup

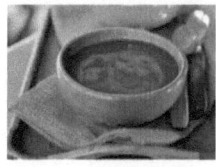

This vibrant soup is a source of anti-oxidants, which can keep cancer at bay!

Ingredients

- 1 ½ medium beets, peeled and cut into halves
- ½ teaspoon olive oil
- ½ cup chopped onion
- ½ medium potato, peeled and cut into halves
- 4 teaspoons reduced-fat sour cream
- 2 cups chicken broth, low- sodium and fat free
- ¼ teaspoon salt
- ½ bay leaf
- ½ teaspoon lemon juice
- 1/8 teaspoon freshly ground black pepper
- 1 cup water

Method

1. In a Dutch oven, heat the olive oil over medium high heat. Sauté the chopped onions in the heated oil till they turn become tender. Add the chicken broth, potatoes, beets, bay leaf and water and stir well.

2. Sprinkle the salt and pepper on top of the mixture and combine well. Bring the mixture to a boil and let it simmer for around twenty minutes. This will give the beets and potatoes enough time to become tender. Remove the bay leaf from the mixture and puree the soup with the help of a blender.

3. Heat the pureed soup over low heat for around five minutes. Remove the pan from the heat and add the lemon juice to the soup. Add in the sour cream and stir well before transferring it to the serving bowls.

Tips/Notes

Beets are the natural source of a nutrient called Betaine, which helps in the protection of the million cells in our body. Betaine also possesses anti-inflammatory properties and can help in the protection of internal organs. Beets are a rich source of Vitamin C which helps in improving your immune system.

6. Sweet and Sour Chicken

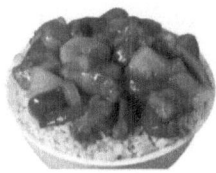

This exquisite chicken delicacy can not only be refreshing to your palette but also replenish your body with nutrients like selenium, niacin and vitamin B6.

Ingredients

- 4 chicken breasts, skinless and boneless (cut into chunks)
- 2 red peppers, seeded and cut into chunks
- 3 tablespoons malt vinegar
- tablespoons tomato ketchup
- 4 tablespoons dark Muscovado sugar
- 1 small onion, chopped coarsely
- 2 garlic cloves, finely crushed
- 100 g sugar snap peas, sliced roughly
- Handful of roasted cashews
- 227 g pineapple, chopped

Method

1. Take a large microwave friendly bowl. Add the chopped chicken, peppers, onion to the bowl. Add the ketchup, vinegar, garlic and sugar to it and mix all the ingredients well. Microwave it on high heat for around ten minutes. Remove the bowl from the microwave once the sauce starts sizzling. Add the pineapple pieces and sugar snap peas to the bowl and mix well.

2. Heat the bowl in the microwave for another three minutes for the chicken to get cooked completely. Remove the bowl from the microwave and keep it aside for a few minutes. Garnish with the roasted cashews and serve hot.

7. Vegetarian Stuffed Mushrooms

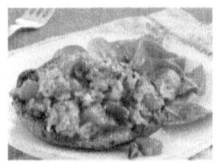

Being an excellent source of vitamin D, this light snack can be quite an appetizer!

Ingredients

- 4 large Portobello mushroom caps
- 1 ½ cups chopped tomatoes
- 2 teaspoons olive oil
- 1/3 cup chopped Kalamata olives
- ½ cup (4 ounces) shredded Fontina cheese
- 1 cup fresh whole-grain breadcrumbs
- 1 ½ tablespoons balsamic vinegar
- ¼ cup chopped fresh chives
- ½ teaspoon freshly ground black pepper
- ¼ teaspoon coarse sea salt

Method

1. Preheat the oven to about 400 degrees. Arrange the mushroom caps neatly on a rimmed baking sheet in such a fashion that the gill side is up. Drizzle with vinegar and olive oil and season the mushrooms with ¼ teaspoon of the freshly ground black pepper and salt. Bake the mushrooms in the oven for around ten minutes until they turn tender.

2. In a medium sized bowl, mix the tomato, chives, olives, breadcrumbs and cheese. Season the mixture with the remaining black pepper and mix. Stuff the mushroom caps with the tomato mixture and bake them for another ten minutes till they turn light brown in color. Serve hot.

Tips/Notes

Mushrooms are perhaps the only vegetable that is rich in vitamin D. Mushrooms contain a compound called lectins, which can prevent the formation and growth of cancer causing cells in our body. Regular intake of mushrooms helps in keeping the blood glucose levels normal.

8. Jam Biscuits

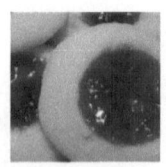

These healthy biscuits can be an easy alternative to your calorie-laden chocolate cookies and treats!

Ingredients

- 100 g caster sugar
- 200 g self-rising flour
- 100 g butter
- 4 tablespoons raspberry jam
- 1 egg, lightly beaten

Method

1. Pre-heat the oven to 190 degrees Celsius. Take a large bowl. Add the flour, butter and sugar to the bowl and mix them well till they attain the texture of breadcrumbs. Add in the beaten egg and combine well till it becomes dough-like. Sprinkle some flour on top of the kitchen counter. Using your hands, shape the dough into a tube. Cut the tube into small and thick slices and arrange the slices on a baking sheet.

2. Use a spoon to create a tiny indentation in the middle of the slices and add about a teaspoon of the jam to each slice. Bake it in the oven for around fifteen minutes until they turn golden. Cool the biscuits on a wire rack and serve.

9. Scallops in Parchment with Fennel, Tomatoes, and Olives

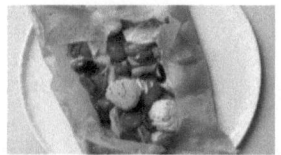

A regular intake of scallops can improve our metabolism and can keep different kinds of cancers at bay. Say no to colon cancer with this refreshing dish!

Ingredients

- 2 small fennel heads, cored and sliced thinly
- 1-pound sea scallops
- 1 tablespoon extra-virgin olive oil
- ½ cup pitted kalamata olives, cut into halves
- 1-pint grape tomatoes, cut into halves

- ¼ cup dry white wine
- ¼ teaspoon kosher salt
- 1 clove garlic, sliced thinly
- ¼ teaspoon black pepper

Method

1. Pre-heat the oven to 375 degrees. Take four 16x12 inch pieces of parchment and fold them into half. Unfold the parchment on top of two baking sheets. Neatly arrange the fennel, olives, scallops, tomatoes and garlic on half of each parchment and season them well with salt and pepper. Drizzle with olive oil and white wine. Fold the parchments and crimp the edges in such a fashion that they are sealed.

2. Bake them in the oven for around fifteen to twenty minutes until the scallops are cooked. The packets will puff up when the scallops are cooked through. Transfer the parchment packets to the serving plates and cut them open!

Tips/Notes

Fennel is an important source of all the nutrients that help in maintaining the health of the bones in our body. It is rich in phosphorous, magnesium, calcium, vitamin K, zinc and manganese.

Regular intake of fennel is a proven cure for hypertension owing to the presence of nutrients like potassium, magnesium and calcium.

Selenium, a rare mineral, is found abundant in fennel which is capable of detoxifying any cancer inducing compounds in the body.

10. Thai Prawn Curry

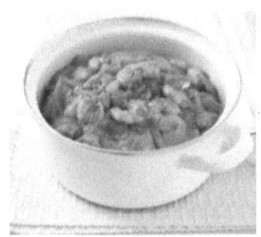

This protein rich prawn delicacy can be an interesting and healthy alternative for red meat, thereby reducing your intake of saturated fat.

Ingredients

- 400 g raw and frozen prawns
- 1 onion, finely chopped
- 1 tablespoon vegetable oil
- 1 teaspoon fresh root ginger
- 400 g tomatoes, finely chopped
- 2 teaspoon Thai red curry paste
- 50 g coconut cream
- Coriander, finely chopped
- Water

Method

1. Pour the oil into a medium sized saucepan and heat it. Add the chopped onion and ginger to the pan and cook it for a few minutes till the onions turn soft. Stir in the red curry paste and let it cook for another minute. Add the chopped tomatoes and the coconut cream to the pan and mix well. Bring the mixture to a boil.

2. Let the mixture simmer for around five minutes. Pour in some water if the consistency of the curry is too thick. Add the prawns to the pan and let it cook for about ten minutes. Garnish with the chopped cilantro and serve hot.

11. Spicy Falafel

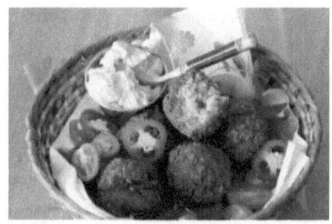

Light and packed with flavors, this falafel is a rich source of fiber and protein! It is not only a healthy option for people allergic to gluten but also helps in improving your metabolism.

Ingredients

- 800 g chickpeas, washed and drained
- 2 small onions, finely chopped
- 4 tablespoons sunflower or vegetable oil

- 2 garlic cloves, crushed
- 2 teaspoons ground coriander
- 2 teaspoons ground cumin
- 2 eggs, beaten
- Handful of fresh parsley, finely chopped
- Pita bread

Method

1. Heat two tablespoons of the oil over low heat in a large pan. Add the chopped garlic and onions to the pan and fry it for around five minutes till the onions turn soft. Take a large bowl. Add the chickpeas, cumin and coriander to it and mix well. Add the fried onions and garlic to the mixture and combine well.

2. Add the chopped parsley and the eggs to the mixture next. With the help of your hands, combine the mixture well. Shape the mixture into 12 evenly shaped balls. Flatten the balls into patties. Pour the remaining oil into the pan and heat it. Fry the patties in the pan over medium heat. Cook each side for around three minutes for them to turn golden brown. Serve them hot with some pita bread.

Tips/Notes

Chickpeas are proven to have reduced the risk of both Type-1 and Type-2 diabetes. They are a source of all the nutrients that help in maintaining the health of the bones in our body. It is rich in phosphorous, magnesium, calcium, vitamin K, zinc and manganese. Chickpeas can lower the amount of LDL (low density lipoprotein) cholesterol in the blood.

12. Parmesan Spring Chicken

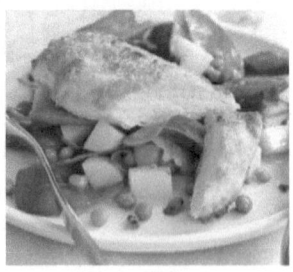

This energy-packed chicken dish can not only be an interesting choice for dinner but also helps in the effective functioning of your digestive system.

Ingredients

- 4 chicken breasts, boneless and skinless
- tablespoons finely grated parmesan cheese
- 1 egg white
- 400 g potatoes, cubed
- 1 tablespoon white wine vinegar
- 140 g frozen peas
- 2 teaspoons olive oil
- Handful of baby spinach leaves
- Salt, to taste
- Pepper, to taste
- Water

Method

1. Heat grill to medium. Arrange a foil over the grill pan. Beat the egg white well in a small plate and season it with salt and pepper. Place the parmesan cheese in another plate. Dip the chicken breasts in the egg white first and then in the cheese. Cook the chicken breasts on the grill for around ten minutes till they turn brown and crisp. In the meantime, add some water to a large pot. Boil the potatoes in the pot for around ten minutes.

2. At the end of seven minutes, add the peas to the pot. Remove the potatoes and peas from the pot at the end of ten minutes. Mix the potatoes, peas, spinach, olive oil, vinegar well. Season the mixture with salt and pepper. Serve the potato mixture with the chicken breasts.

13. Marinated Smoked Salmon with Poppy Seeds

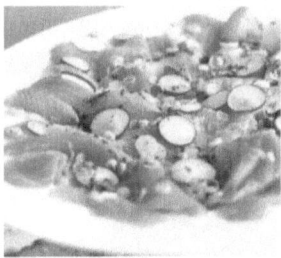

Now replenish the vitamin D content in your body with just a serving of this dish!

Ingredients

- 600 g smoked salmon
- 2 tablespoons poppy seeds, toasted lightly
- 170 g radishes, trimmed and sliced thinly
- Juice from 2 oranges
- Spring onions, sliced finely
- Zest from four oranges
- 4 teaspoons red wine vinegar
- 1 teaspoon sesame oil
- 4 teaspoons olive oil
- Salt, to taste
- Pepper, to taste
- Toasted rye, to serve

Method

1. Add the orange juice, zest, poppy seeds, sesame oil, vinegar, olive oil to a medium sized bowl and whisk them well. Season with pinch of salt and pepper and mix well. Neatly arrange the slices of salmon along with the three fourths of the radishes and spring onions in a large mixing bowl. Pour the dressing over the salmon and the vegetables and mix well with the help of your hands.

2. Allow the salmon to marinate for not more than ten minutes. Arrange the marinated salmon in serving plates. Garnish it with remaining spring onions and radishes. Serve it with the toasted rye.

Tips/Notes

Salmon contains omega-3 fatty acid DHA which helps in the brain functions. Consuming salmon at least twice a week can reduce the risk of macular degeneration which is a chronic eye condition that results in the loss of vision. Being an excellent source of tryptophan, salmon induces sleep! Say goodbye to insomnia with salmon!

14. Garlic & Basil Ciabatta

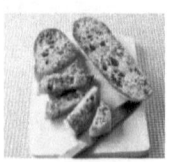

The basil content in this light appetizer can help in dealing with indigestion and has a soothing effect on the stomach!

Ingredients

- 1 small Ciabatta
- 2 garlic cloves, finely crushed
- 2 tablespoons butter, softened
- 1 bunch of basil, finely chopped
- 2 tablespoons grated parmesan
- 1 tablespoon mayonnaise
- Salt, to taste
- Pepper, to taste

Method

1. Heat the grill to high. In a small bowl, mix the butter, mayonnaise and garlic well. Add the chopped basil to the butter mixture and mix well. Season with salt and pepper.

2. Slice the Ciabatta into two halves (lengthwise) and arrange it on a baking tray. Coat the halves with the butter mixture and garnish each half with the grated parmesan cheese. Grill the Ciabatta slices for around three minutes. Serve warm.

15. Tomato and Thyme Cod

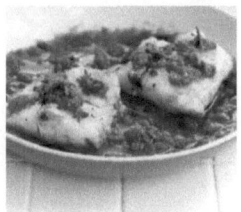

Lower the levels of triglycerides in your blood with just two servings of this dish!

Ingredients

- Cod fillets
- 800 g chopped tomatoes
- 2 onions, finely chopped
- 2 tablespoons olive oil

- 2 teaspoons soft and light brown sugar
- 2 tablespoons soy sauce
- Few sprigs thyme

Method

1. Take a medium sized frying pan and heat the olive oil in it. Add the chopped onions to the pan and fry it for around five to eight minutes till they turn golden brown. Add the chopped tomatoes, thyme, sugar and soy sauce to the pan next and mix well. Bring the mixture to a boil.

2. Let it simmer for around five minutes before you add the cod fillets to the pan. Let the fillets cook in the mixture for around ten minutes till they turn flaky. Remove it from the heat and serve hot.

Tips/Notes

Cod is rich in selenium and vitamin B12 which can prevent the formation of cancer inducing cells in the body. Being a rich source of omega-3 fatty acids, cod is proven to have improved the functions of the heart. It contains a nutrient called niacin which can help in lowering the high levels of cholesterol in the blood.

16. Pan-Fried Scallops with Lime & Coriander

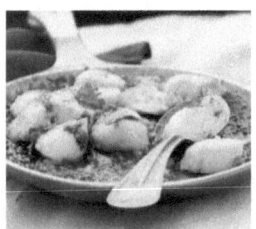

Consumption of scallops at least thrice a month can help you battle against ischemic stroke which is generally caused by the lack of blood supply to the brain! Begin these battles with this light dish!

Ingredients

- to 8 scallops
- Juice from half a lime
- 1 tablespoon olive oil
- 1 teaspoon chopped red chili

- 2 large garlic cloves, finely chopped
- Salt, to taste
- Pepper, to taste
- Handful of fresh coriander, coarsely chopped

Method

1. Take a medium sized frying pan. Heat the olive oil in the pan. Fry the scallops in the heated oil for around one minute or until they golden. At the end of one minute, flip them to the other side.

2. Add the chopped garlic and red chili to the pan and cook for another minute. Pour the lemon juice over the scallops. Season the cooked scallops with salt and pepper. Garnish with the chopped coriander and serve hot.

17. Creamed Spinach

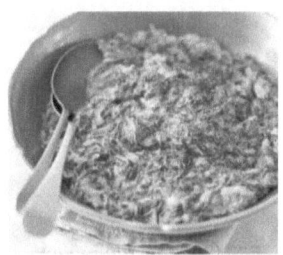

This anti-oxidant rich soup is capable of keeping asthma and other respiratory issues at bay owing to the presence of beta-carotene.

Ingredients

- 400 g spinach
- 1 small onion, finely chopped
- 200 ml full-fat milk
- 2 tablespoons plain flour
- 100 ml single cream
- 25 g butter
- fresh nutmeg, for grating

Method

1. Take a medium sized saucepan and melt the butter in it. Add the onions to the pan and cook it for around five minutes till they soften.

Add the flour to the pan and mix well. Whisk in the milk slowly and cook it for five minutes till the sauce reaches a thick consistency.

2. In the meantime, arrange the spinach in a colander. Pour some boiling water over the spinach until the leaves become wilted. Remove the spinach from the colander and drain out any excess liquid. Chop it coarsely and add it to the sauce. Add the cream to the pan at this stage. Gently heat it for another minute and transfer it to serving bowls. Grate some nutmeg over each bowl and serve.

Tips/Notes

Spinach is rich in alpha-lipoic acid, an anti-oxidant that can lower the blood glucose levels and help in the prevention of diabetes. The high potassium content in spinach helps in lowering high levels of blood pressure. Being a natural source of vitamin A, spinach helps in the growth of various tissues in the body.

18. Scones with Clotted Cream and Jam

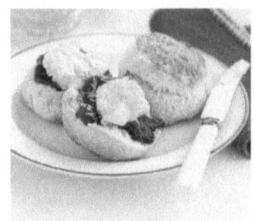

This low-calorie version of scones can be the ideal breakfast option!

Ingredients

- 350 g self-rising flour, plus more for dusting
- ¼ teaspoon salt
- 1 teaspoon baking powder
- 85 g butter, cut in 1-inch cubes
- 3 tablespoons castor sugar
- 175 ml milk
- Vanilla extract
- Lemon juice
- 1 beaten egg, for glaze
- Jam, to serve
- Clotted cream, to serve

Method

1. Preheat the oven to 220 degrees Celsius. Take a large bowl. Add the flour, salt and baking powder to the bowl and mix them well. Add the butter to the mixture and combine them to resemble breadcrumbs. Add the sugar to the mixture and combine well. Heat the milk in a jug in the microwave for around thirty seconds till it turns warm. Add the vanilla and lemon juice to the warm milk and keep it aside. Mix the flour mixture and the milk mixture together till it turns into dough.

2. Dust the kitchen counter with some flour and work the dough on the powdered surface. Shape the dough into a smooth circle. Cut out 8 scones from the dough and brush each scone with the beaten egg. Line a baking tray with parchment paper and arrange the scones on it. Bake the tray in the oven for around ten minutes till they turn golden in color. Top each scone with jam and clotted cream and serve.

19. Cheese, Leek and Potato Tortilla

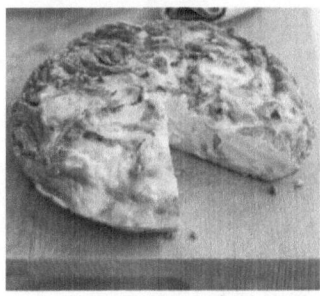

Despite being loaded sinfully with cheese, this is quite low on calories! The leeks used in the dish are rich in Lutein and Zeaxanthin that promote healthy eyesight.

Ingredients

- 225 g potatoes cooked and cooled
- 1 leek, thinly sliced
- Eggs
- 85 g cheddar
- 1 tablespoon sage, finely chopped
- Butter
- Salt, to taste
- Pepper, to taste

Method

1. Melt the butter in a medium sized frying pan. Add the leek to the pan and cook it for about five minutes. As the leeks are getting cooked, cut the potatoes into smaller pieces.

2. In a small bowl, beat the eggs well. Season with salt and pepper and add the cheese and sage to it. Mix it all well. Now add the potatoes to the pan followed by the egg mixture. Cook the mixture on low heat for around ten minutes until it is set. Place the mixture under a hot grill and cook them for another two minutes. Slice it into evenly shaped wedges and serve.

Tips/Notes

The rich iron content present in leeks can keep anemia at bay. Leek possesses both anti-inflammatory as well anti-septic properties and an effective cure for arthritis and gout. Owing to the high content of volatile oils, leek is capable of inducing a balsamic action on the respiratory tract thereby help in curing hay.

20. Couscous with Garlicky Grilled Tilapia

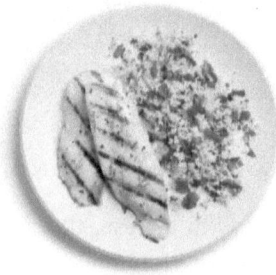

Marinate fish in olive oil, garlic and lemon juice to infuse it with the right flavors before grilling.

Ingredients

- 2 tablespoons chopped and sun-dried tomatoes
- 1 tablespoon chopped fresh flat-leaf parsley
- 1 cup couscous split lengthwise
- 4 6-ounce tilapia fillets
- Black pepper and chopped kosher salt
- 2 cloves garlic
- 1 tablespoon olive oil

- Plus wedges for serving
- 2 tablespoons fresh lemon juice

Method

1. Combine lemon juice, garlic, olive oil, ¼ teaspoon pepper and ½ teaspoon salt. Add tilapia and toss to coat and marinate it for 10 minutes. Meanwhile, cook couscous according to package directions.

2. Remove it from heat and stir in sun-dried tomatoes and parsley. Heat the grill to high heat. Grill the fish on oiled grate until it's cooked through for about 2 minutes per side.

Tips/Notes

Tilapia contains an impressive amount of proteins and makes for over 15% of the daily requirement per serving.

21. Asparagus and Bulgur with Lemony Baked Salmon

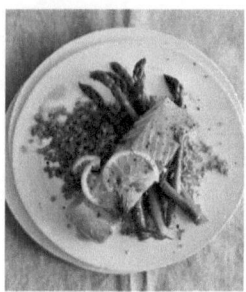

This is one of the low calories-healthy recipes. It's a snap to prepare—all the ingredients cook together in the same dish in an oven.

Ingredients

- 2 tablespoons chopped fresh dill olive oil
- 1 very thinly sliced lemon
- Skinless salmon fillet (1 1/4 pounds) cut into 4 pieces
- (1 bunch), 1-pound asparagus trimmed
- Black pepper
- Chicken broth kosher salt or 1 1/2 cups low-sodium vegetable
- ½ teaspoon salt
- 1 cup bulgur

Method

1. Heat the oven to 375° F. Combine broth, bulgur, and ¼ teaspoon salt and pepper each in a shallow baking dish. Lay the asparagus in a single layer top and place salmon on top. Season the salmon with ¼ teaspoon pepper, 1/4 teaspoon salt and top with lemon.

2. Cover the baking dish tightly using foil and let it bake for about 25 minutes or until the asparagus and bulgur are cooked and tender. Serve the salmon with the asparagus and bulgur. Drizzle with the oil and sprinkle with the dill.

Tips/Notes

Salmon is an excellent source of selenium, vitamin D and vitamin B12. It's a great source of omega-3 fatty acids and is rich in an antioxidant amino acid taurine.

22. Barbecued Chipotle-Marinated Pork Sandwiches

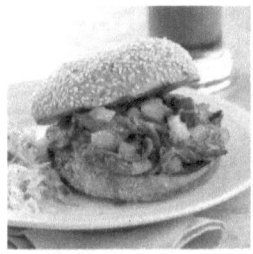

Your favorite barbecue sauce and smoky grilled onion this recipe into a mouthwatering pulled pork sandwich.

Ingredients

- 1/3 cup barbecue sauce (prepared)
- 2 whole-wheat horizontally split buns
- 1 teaspoon canola oil
- 1 yellow onion, sliced into 1/2-inch-thick rounds
- Pork tenderloin trimmed (8 ounces)
- 1/4 teaspoon freshly ground pepper
- 1/4 teaspoon salt
- 1/2 teaspoon ground cumin
- 1 teaspoon dried oregano
- 1 clove minced garlic

- 1 teaspoon adobo sauce
- 1 chipotle chilled in adobo sauce
- 1 tablespoon red-wine vinegar
- 3 tablespoons lime juice
- 1/2 cup orange juice

Method

1. Combine chipotle, vinegar, lime juice, orange juice, pepper, salt, cumin, oregano, garlic and sauce in a mini food processor or blender. Process or blend until the mixture becomes relatively smooth and chipotle is chopped. Pour it into a sealable bag and add pork. Seal and squeeze out excess air from the bag. Marinate until it turns to coat and refrigerate it. Heat the grill to high heat and remove the pork from the marinade. Discard marinade and grill the pork, turning it frequently for about 15 minutes.

2. Transfer it to a cutting board and let it rest for about 5 minutes before slicing. Meanwhile, brush oil with onion and grill until soft and lightly browned, turning once in 5 minutes. Place it on a cutting board and allow it to cool. Toast buns lightly in the pan or on the grill. Cut the onion and transfer it to a larger bowl. Shred the pork with two forks and add it to the bowl. Add sauce and mix. Divide the pork between the buns.

Tips/Notes

Pork is rich in protein, vitamin B (B6, B12, niacin and thiamin). It's also low in fat and plays a role in metabolism.

23. Pecorino & Ravioli with Arugula

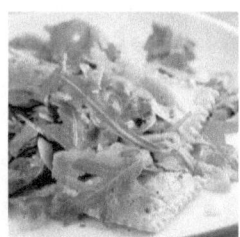

Elevate the shaved pecorino, frozen ravioli, shallots, sizzled garlic and fresh arugula. Serve it with a light bodied red wine such as pinot noir. You may also serve with whole grain baguette.

Ingredients

- 1/2 cup parmesan cheese or shaved Pecorino Romano
- 6 cups arugula
- Freshly ground pepper
- 1 teaspoon Dijon mustard
- 3 tablespoons red-wine vinegar
- 2 large sliced shallots
- 1/4 cup olive oil
- 1/2 teaspoon kosher salt
- 1 large minced clove garlic
- 1 pound frozen or fresh cheese ravioli, preferably whole-wheat

Method

1. Bring a large bowl of water to boil and cook ravioli for about 10 minutes, until tender or according to the package directions. Meanwhile, add salt to garlic and mash into a paste using the back of a spoon or a chef's knife. Heat the olive oil over medium heat in a small skillet.

2. Add shallots, garlic paste and cook, stirring occasionally, until it begins to turn brown (about 3 minutes). Stir in mustard, pepper and vinegar and remove from heat. Drain the ravioli properly and place it in a larger bowl Toss with arugula and the dressing. Sprinkle with cheese and serve.

Tips/Notes

Arugula has very few calories and tons of flavors. Its helps maintain healthy weight without having to sacrificing tasty foods.

24. Chops au Poivre

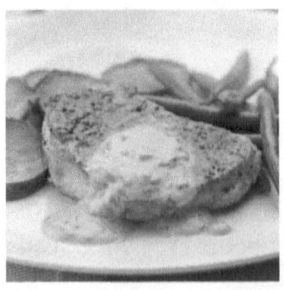

This recipe combines the rich creamy brandy sauce with pepper crusted pork chops. Serve it with green beans and roasted sweet potato slices.

Ingredients

- 1/4 cup reduced-fat sour cream
- 1/2 cup brandy
- 1 medium minced shallot
- 2 tablespoons olive oil
- 3 tablespoons all-purpose flour
- 1/2-inch-thick, trimmed boneless pork chops
- 1/2 (divided) teaspoon salt
- 1 teaspoon black pepper

Method

1. Combine 1/4 teaspoon salt and pepper in a small bowl. Mix and pat it onto both sides of each pork chop. Place the all-purpose flour in a dish; dredge the chops in the flour, shaking off excesses. Turn the heat to medium-high and eat oil in a large skillet. Add the chops and then reduce the heat down to medium. Cook until browned for 2-3 minutes per side and transfer to a tent and plate with foil to keep warm.

2. Turn the heat to medium low and add shallot to the pan. Stir until softened for about 2 minutes. Add the brandy and cook, scraping and stirring up browned bits until most of the liquid evaporates (about 2 minutes). Remove it from heat and stir in the remaining 1/4 teaspoon salt and sour cream. Serve with the sauce.

Tips/Notes

The sweetly shaped shallots offer a special flavor to your meals—plus a healthy helping of antioxidants.

25. Balsamic Onion Quesadillas & Turkey

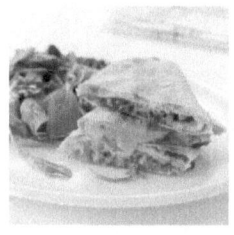

This is not the traditional quesadilla you are used to. It features cheddar cheese, deli turkey as well as onions marinated in balsamic vinegar. Serve with a tossed salad and sautéed vegetables for a quick meal.

Ingredients

- 8 slices (8 ounces) deli turkey, (preferably smoked)
- 1 cup Cheddar cheese, shredded sharp
- 4 10-inch whole-wheat tortillas
- 1/4 cup balsamic vinegar
- 1 thinly sliced red onion

Method

1. Combine vinegar and onion in a bowl. Marinate it for about 5 minutes. Drain and reserve the vinegar for another use, for example salad dressing. Warm the 2 tortillas in a nonstick skillet over medium heat for about 1 minute and flip. Pull the tortillas up the edges of the baking to avoid overlapping.

2. Working with 1/2 of each tortilla, sprinkle 1/4 of the cheese and cover with 2 slices of the turkey. Top with the onion and fold the tortillas in half, flattening them gently using a spatula. Cook until the cheese begins to melt for about 2 minutes. Flip it and cook for about 2 minutes or until the other side turns golden. Transfer it to a plate and cover to keep warm. Prepare 2 more quesadillas using the remaining ingredients.

Tips/Notes

Olive oil and balsamic vinegar both contain anti-oxidants that may lower the risk of heart related diseases. Olive contains vitamin K and E while Balsamic vinegar is low in calories and helps deal with blood sugar levels.

26. Black Beans with Southwestern Salad

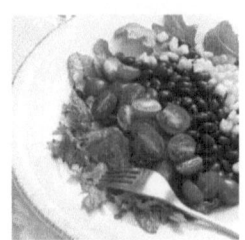

In this recipe, we top black beans with top salad greens, grape tomatoes, sweet corn, bringing it all together with a tangy avocado-lime dressing for a one-of-a-kind Mexican salad. You can prepare this salad as a take-along lunch. To avoid the salad greens from becoming soggy, pack salad toppings, greens and dressing in separate bowls and toss them together prior to serving.

Ingredients

- 1/2 cup grape tomatoes
- 1/2 cup frozen (thawed) or corn kernels, fresh
- 1/2 cup black beans, cooked or canned (rinsed)
- 3 cups mixed greens
- 1/2 teaspoon salt
- 1/2 teaspoon sugar
- 1 tablespoon lime juice
- 1 clove quartered garlic
- 2 chopped scallions
- 1/2 cup nonfat plain yogurt
- 3/4 cup packed fresh cilantro
- 1/2 ripe avocado

Method

1. Place cilantro, yogurt, avocado, garlic, lime juice, scallions, salt and sugar in a blender; blend until smooth. Place the salad greens in a salad bowl and toss with 2 tablespoons of the dressing and refrigerate the rest of the dressing. Top the salad greens with tomatoes, corn and black beans.

Tips/Notes

Just like other legumes, black beans are prized for their fiber and protein content. They also contain minerals and other key vitamins known to benefit human health.

27. Cornmeal-Crusted Chicken Nuggets with Blackberry Mustard

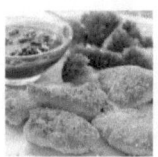

Tossing cornmeal with chicken tenders gives the chicken nuggets great crunch without having to deep fry. Blackberries combined with mustard (or raspberries if you prefer) make for the most delicious savory dipping sauce. Serve with carrots and broccoli.

Ingredients

- 1 tablespoon olive oil
- 3 tablespoons cornmeal
- 1/4 teaspoon freshly ground pepper
- 1/2 teaspoon salt
- 1-pound chicken tenders, split into half crosswise
- 2 teaspoons honey
- 1 1/2 tablespoons whole-grain mustard
- 1 cup fresh finely chopped blackberries

Method

1. Mash the blackberries (or raspberries, if you prefer), honey and mustard in a bowl until it turns chunky. Sprinkle salt and pepper on the chicken tenders. Place the cornmeal in a bowl and add toss and chicken to coat. Discard cornmeal leftovers.

2. In a large nonstick skillet, heat olive oil. Turn the heat to medium and cook the chicken, occasionally turning it once or twice until it's cooked through and browned (about 6-8) minutes in total (thinner nuggets will cook faster that thicker ones). Serve the chicken nuggets with blackberry mustard.

Tips/Notes

Blackberries contain only 62 calories in one cup and are rich in vitamin C and bioflavonoids. Did you know that the black blue color ensures they have the highest levels of antioxidants?

28. Greek Salad with Sardines

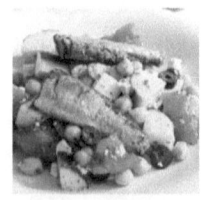

The tangy, fresh elements of Greek salad—cucumber, feta, tomato, lemony vinaigrette and olives—pair perfectly well with rich tasting sardines. Find sardines that still have skin and bones (edible) since they contain close to four times the level of calcium as boneless, skinless sardines. If you are lucky to find fresh sardines in a supermarket, you may opt to try them in place of canned sardines. Dredge them lightly in pepper-and-salt-seasoned flour and sauté in olive oil.

Ingredients

- 2 4-ounce cans sardines (with bones), packed in water or olive oil, drained
- 2 tablespoons sliced Kalamata olives
- 1/4 cup red onion (thinly sliced)
- 1/3 cup crumbled feta cheese
- 1 1/5-ounce cans chickpeas, rinsed
- 1 English cucumber, split into large chunks
- 3 tomatoes sliced into large chunks
- 1/2 teaspoon freshly ground pepper
- 2 teaspoons dried oregano
- 1 clove minced garlic
- 2 tablespoons olive oil
- 3 tablespoons lemon juice

Method

1. Whisk oil, garlic, lemon juice, pepper and oregano in a bowl and combine them well. Add chickpeas, feta, cucumber, olives, and onions; gently toss to mix. Serve and top with sardines.

Tips/Notes

Sardines contain high levels of healthy unsaturated fat which helps lower cholesterol levels and minimize the risk of heart related diseases.

29. Troy's Hana-Style Sauce with Ginger-Steamed Fish

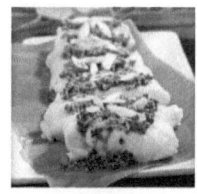

This recipe features the shoyu sauce that contains garlic, sesame and fresh ginger. This recipe can be prepared with onaga, a red snapper for added flavor and sweetness. Serve with green papaya salad and steamed brown rice.

Ingredients

For the Fish

- 6 5-ounce portions halibut, striped bass, or any white fish

For the Sauce

- 2-3 scallions, thinly sliced
- 1/4 cup reduced-sodium soy sauce
- 2 tablespoons sesame oil (toasted)
- 2 tablespoons canola or grapeseed oil
- 1/4 cup sesame seeds
- 1/4 cup garlic
- Fresh ginger

Method

1. To prepare the fish: Bring 1-2 inches of water to boil in a bowl that's big enough to hold two-tier bamboo steamer. In case you do not have a steamer, improvise it by setting mugs upside down in a large bowl. Rest a heatproof plate in each steamer baskets. Onto each plate of fresh ginger top, add 3 portions of fish. Stack each basket, cover and set over boiling water.

2. Steam the fish for about 7 minutes per inch of thickness. To make sauce, combine minced ginger, sesame seeds and garlic in a bowl. Put canola oil (or grapeseed oil) in a skillet and heat over medium-heat. Add the ginger mixture, stirring for 1 minute or until fragrant. Add the sesame oil and wait until the mixture gets hot. Then add soy sauce and cook for one more minute. Be careful when adding soy sauce, it will splatter a bit. Put the fish in a deep platter. Discard the ginger slices and pour the sauce over the fish. Garnish with scallions.

Tips/Notes

Ginger present in this recipe has Gingerol, an ingredient that has very powerful medicinal properties for the treatments of nausea, particularly morning sickness. It also reduces muscle soreness and pain.

30. Cube Steak with Mushroom-Sherry Sauce

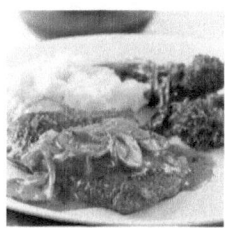

The reason why most people like cube steak is because it's inexpensive and cooks quickly. It's a tougher cut of meat pounded to make it tender. Cube steak makes for a great low-calorie weeknight meal.

Ingredients

- 2 tablespoons reduced-fat sour cream
- 1/2 cup reduced-sodium beef broth
- 1/2 cup dry sherry
- 1/4 teaspoon dried thyme or 1 teaspoon chopped fresh thyme
- 1 tablespoon all-purpose flour
- 1 large thinly sliced shallot
- 2 1/2 cups sliced mushrooms
- 2 tablespoons olive oil, divided
- 1/2 teaspoon salt
- 3/4 teaspoon freshly ground pepper, divided
- 4 4-ounce cube steaks

Method

1. Sprinkle cube steaks with salt and 1/2 teaspoon pepper. Heat 1 tablespoon olive oil in a large nonskilled over medium heat. Add steaks, turning once. Cook until through or browned (about 2 minutes) per side. Cook in 2 batches if desired and transfer the cube steaks to another plate and cover to keep warm.

2. Add the remaining olive oil to the pan and add shallot, mushroom and the remaining pepper; cook and stir until the mushrooms turn golden brown for about 5 minutes. Sprinkle with flour and cook for 1-minute stirring occasionally. Add sherry, broth and thyme and bring to boil while stirring until its thick enough to coat, about 3 minutes. Remove from heat and stir in sour cream. Return the cube steaks to the pan. Turn to coat and serve with the sauce.

Tips/Notes

Mushrooms contain high levels of B vitamins such as folate, riboflavin, pantothenic acid, thiamine and niacin and minerals; selenium and iron that may be difficult to obtain in most foods.

31. Marmalade Chicken

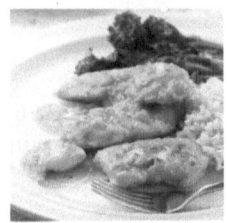

Freshly grated orange zest and orange marmalade make a perfectly delicious with chicken tenders. Best when served brown rice.

Ingredients

- 1 teaspoon freshly grated orange zest
- 2 large minced shallots
- 6 teaspoons olive oil, divided
- 1/4 teaspoon freshly ground pepper
- 1/2 teaspoon kosher salt
- 1-pound chicken tenders
- 1 teaspoon cornstarch
- 1 teaspoon Dijon mustard
- 2 tablespoons orange marmalade
- 2 tablespoons red-wine vinegar
- 1 cup reduced-sodium chicken broth

Method

1. Whisk vinegar, marmalade, broth, cornstarch and mustard in a medium bowl. Sprinkle with pepper and salt. Transfer the mixture to a plate and cover with foil to keep warm. Heat the 4 teaspoons olive oil in a large skillet over medium-high heat. Add the chicken and cook for about 2 minutes or until golden. Add the remaining 2 teaspoons olive oil and shallots to the pan. Add shallots and cook.

2. Stir until browned (about 30 seconds) then whisk the broth mixture and add it to the pan. Bring to a simmer while scraping up any

browned bits. Maintain the simmer by turning the heat to medium. Cook until the sauce is slightly thickened and reduced, 1-2 minutes. Add the chicken and cook, occasionally turning it until the chicken is totally heated through (about 1 minute). Remove from the heat and add orange zest. Stir and serve.

Tips/Notes

Chicken provides a good supply of essential vitamins, protein and minerals. It helps in weight loss and cholesterol control.

32. Creamy Piccata Sauce with Poached Salmon

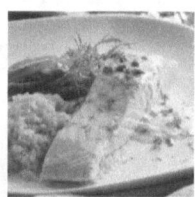

Easy poached salmon is delicious with creamy piccata sauce. Prepare it and serve with roasted asparagus or snow peas and brown rice or whole grain like quinoa.

Ingredients

- 1 tablespoon chopped fresh dill
- 1/4 teaspoon salt
- 1/4 cup reduced-fat sour cream
- 4 teaspoons rinsed capers
- 2 tablespoons lemon juice
- 1 large minced shallot
- 2 teaspoons olive oil
- 1 cup dry white wine, divided
- 1-pound center-split salmon fillet, preferably skinned and split into 4 portions

Method

1. Place salmon in a large skillet and add 1/2 wine. Add enough water to cover the salmon. Turn heat to high heat and bring to boil. Reduce to a simmer and turn the salmon over. Cook for about 5 minutes and remove from heat.

2. Meanwhile, turn heat to medium-high and heat oil in a medium skillet. Add shallot and stir for about 30 seconds or until fragrant. Add the other 1/2 wine and boil for 1 minute. Stir in capers and lemon juice for 2 minutes. Remove from heat and stir in salt and sour cream. Top the salmon with the sauce, garnish with dill and serve.

Tips/Notes

Each tablespoon of capers contains just 2 calories. It adds vibrant and bold flavor to your meals and contain mustard oil. Few capers impart an incredibly big taste to your meals.

33. Pepita-Lime Butter with Salmon

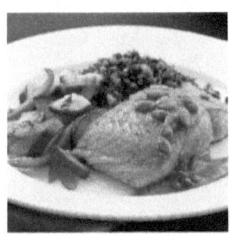

Chili powder, Pepita and lime juice give the salmon a Mexican flair. Serve with steamed vegetables and wild rice.

Ingredients

- 1/4 teaspoon freshly ground pepper
- 1/2 teaspoon salt
- 1-pound salmon fillet preferably skinned and split into 4 portions
- 1/4 teaspoon chili powder
- 2 tablespoons lime juice
- 1/2 teaspoon lime zest (freshly grated)
- 1 tablespoon butter
- 2 tablespoons unsalted Pepita

Method

1. Toast Pepita. Place lime zest, butter, chili powder and lime juice in a bowl. Coat nonstick skillet with cooking spray and place it over medium heat.

2. Sprinkle with pepper and salt. Add it to the pan and cook until just cooked through or browned, 2-5 minutes per side. Now remove from

the heat. Place the salmon in a plate and add butter-lime mixture to the hot pan. Stir until the butter melts completely. Serve the salmon and top with the sauce.

Tips/Notes

Pepita are simply pumpkin seeds. They contain healthy fats as well as fiber, potassium, protein and zinc.

34. Moo Shu Vegetables

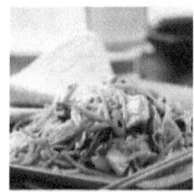

This is a vegetarian version of the classic Chinese stir fry known as Moo Shu. It uses shredded vegetables to cut down on the total preparation time. Serve with extra hoisin, Asian hot sauce and warm whole-wheat tortillas.

Ingredients

- 2 tablespoons hoisin sauce
- 1 tablespoon rice vinegar
- 1 tablespoon soy sauce (reduced sodium)
- 1 bunch sliced and scallions, divided
- 2 cups mung bean sprouts
- 1 1/2-ounce bag shredded mixed vegetables, e.g. "broccoli slaw" or "rainbow salad"
- 2 cloves minced garlic
- 2 teaspoons minced fresh ginger
- 4 large eggs, lightly beaten
- 3 teaspoons toasted sesame oil, divided

Method

1. Turn heat to medium. Heat 1 tablespoon of sesame oil in a large nonstick skillet. Stir in the eggs and cook until set for 2minutes. Transfer to a plate. Wipe the pan clean and heat the remaining 2 tablespoons sesame oil over medium heat. Add garlic and ginger. Cook while stirring until fragrant and softened for 1 minute.

2. Add bean sprouts, soy sauce, vinegar, shredded vegetables and half the sliced scallions. Stir well, cook and cover until the vegetable get just tender, about 4 minutes. Add hoisin and reserved eggs. Cook uncovered. Stir well to break up the scrambled eggs for about 2 minutes. Add the remaining scallions and remove from heat.

Tips/Notes

Green onions are also known as scallions or spring onions. They contain healthy compounds including minerals, phytochemicals and vitamins.

35. Cheddar Soup, Broccoli & Cannellini Bean

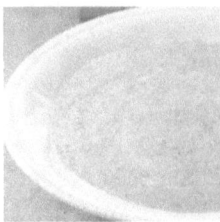

Puree white beans into broccoli soup. This makes it extra creamy so you don't have to add heaps of cheese. Serve with a glass of winter ale and a crunchy whole-grain roll.

Ingredients

- 1 cup shredded extra-sharp Cheddar cheese
- 1/4 teaspoon ground white pepper
- 1/4 teaspoon salt
- 1 14-ounce cans cannellini beans, rinsed
- 6 cups broccoli crowns, chopped and trimmed
- 1 cup water
- 1 14-ounce Can vegetable broth or reduced-sodium chicken broth

Method

1. Over medium heat, bring water and broth to a boil in a medium saucepan. Add broccoli and cook until tender, about 7 minutes. Add beans and stir in pepper and salt until the beans are heated through, about 2 minutes.

2. Transfer half of the mixture to a blender with half the puree and cheese. (Be careful when pureeing hot liquids). Transfer it to a bowl

and repeat the process with the remaining cheese and broccoli mixture. Serve warm.

Tips/Notes

Broccoli contains several important minerals. One of the most important is folate which has been shown to fight cancer.

36. Sweet Potato Hash with Chili-Glazed Pork

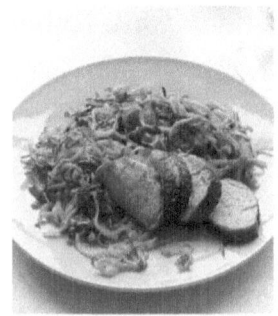

Brush pork with maple syrup when cooking for a mouthwatering glaze.

Ingredients

- 1/5-ounce package chopped baby spinach
- 2 large peeled shallots
- 2 (1 pound) medium sweet potatoes
- 2 tablespoons pure maple syrup
- 1 teaspoon chili powder, black pepper and kosher salt
- 2 tablespoon olive oil
- Chopped hot sauce (optional)
- 1 1/4 pounds pork tenderloin

Method

1. Heat the broiler and place pork on a foil-lined rimmed sheet. Spread with 1 teaspoon olive oil, ¼ teaspoon each salt, chili powder and pepper. Broil while turning and basting with maple syrup.

2. Cook for about 10 minutes and let it rest for 5 minutes before slicing. Meanwhile, grate sweet potatoes on a food processor using a coarse grating disk. In a large nonstick skillet, heat the remaining oil over medium heat. Add shallots and cook while stirring for about 3

minutes. Add sweet potatoes and cook, occasionally stirring until tender for about 10 minutes. Add the spinach, tossing until wilted for 3 minutes. Serve the potatoes and pork with the hot sauce, if desired.

Tips/Notes

Spinach is full of minerals and vitamins. It's incredibly rich in antioxidants and is an impressive source of magnesium, iron, folate, potassium and calcium.

37. Pan Salsa & Chili-Rubbed Steaks

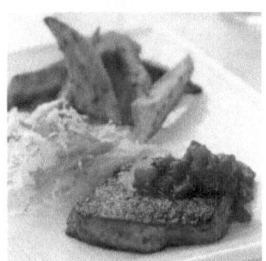

A cut of steak will work just well with this recipe. However, most people tend to love the texture and flavor of rib-eye together with these seasonings. Make sure the steak is thinly cut. Potato fries, vinegar coleslaw and cold ale can round out the meal.

Ingredients

- 1 tablespoon chopped fresh cilantro
- 2 teaspoons lime juice
- 2 diced plum tomatoes
- 1 teaspoon olive oil
- 1/2 teaspoon kosher salt
- 1 teaspoon chili powder
- 1/2-inch-thick steaks, e.g. rib-eye, cut into 2 portions and trimmed of fat

Method

1. Sprinkle both sides of the steak with 1/4 teaspoon salt and chili powder. Turn the heat to medium-high. Now heat oil in a medium skillet and add the steaks. Turn once while cooking for about 1-2 minutes for per side for medium rare.

2. Place the steaks in a plate and cover with foil. Let it rest while you prepare salsa. Add lime juice, tomatoes and the remaining 1/4 teaspoon salt to the pan. Cook while stirring for about 3 minutes or until tomatoes soften properly. Remove from the heat and stir in cilantro as well as any accumulated juices from the steaks. Serve topped with the salsa.

Tips/Notes

One of the major roles of cilantro is that is plays a critical role in blood coagulation thanks to the presence of vitamin K content.

38. Japanese Chicken-Scallion Rice Bowl

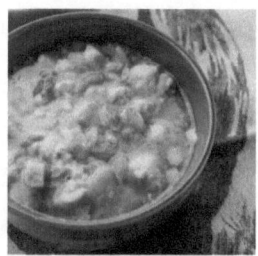

Here is the quintessence of Japanese home cooking. It comes with aromatic, protein-rich broth served with rice. Agreeably, Japanese cooking tends to lean heavily on sugar—for a less traditional taste. You may therefore reduce or omit sugar completely.

Ingredients

- 6 scallions, thinly sliced and trimmed
- 8 ounces skinless, boneless chicken breasts split into 1/2-inch pieces
- 1 large egg
- 2 large egg whites
- 1 tablespoon mirin
- 2 tablespoons reduced-sodium soy sauce
- 1 1/2 tablespoons sugar
- 1 cup reduced-sodium chicken broth
- 1 1/2 cups instant brown rice

Method

1. Prepare instant brown sugar in accordance with the package directions. Add sugar, mirin and soy sauce into a medium saucepan

and pour in the broth. Bring to a boil and turn the heat to medium low. Stir whole egg and egg whites in a bowl and mix well. Now add chicken to the simmering broth. Pour in the egg mixture. Do not stir.

2. Sprinkle the scallions on top. As soon as the egg begins to firm up, after about 4 minutes, stir it with a knife or chopsticks (The chicken will be ready by now). Divide the rice among the 4 bowls and top with chicken mixture.

Tips/Notes

Soy sauce is low in calories with just about 8 calories per tablespoon, 1 gram of carbohydrate and 1 gram of protein.

39. Fettuccine with Shiitake Mushrooms & Basil

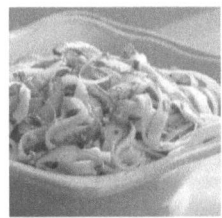

This is one of the fresh-testing whole wheat low calorie pasta recipes I know. The purpose of lemon zest in this recipe is to accent the basil beautifully.

Ingredients

- 1/2 cup chopped fresh basil, divided
- 1/2 cup (1 ounce) Parmesan cheese
- 8 ounces spaghetti or whole-wheat fettuccine
- Freshly ground pepper
- 1/4 teaspoon salt
- 2 tablespoons lemon juice
- 2 teaspoons freshly grated lemon zest
- 2 ounces (1 1/2 cups) shiitake mushrooms, sliced and stemmed
- 3 cloves garlic, minced
- 2 tablespoons extra-virgin olive oil

Method

1. Bring lightly salted water to boil for preparing pasta. Turn the heat to low and heat oil in a large nonstick skillet. Now add garlic and cook,

frequently stirring until fragrant (not browned) for 1 minute. Add mushrooms and turn the heat to medium high. Cook while stirring regularly until lightly browned or tender for about 5 minutes. Stir in lemon juice, salt, lemon zest and pepper. Remove from heat.

2. Meanwhile, prepare pasta, stirring occasionally until just tender for about 10 minutes or according to package directions. Now drain it and reserve 1/2 cup cooking liquid. Add the pasts, 1/4 cup basil, Parmesan, the reserved cooking liquid to the mushrooms in the nonstick skillet. Toss to coat well and serve warm, garnished with the remaining basil.

Tips/Notes

Basil fights the growth of unwanted bacterial growth. Its antibacterial properties are not associated with its unique flavonoids but its volatile oils that are rich in linalool, estragole, cineole, eugenol, myrcene, sabinene and limonene.

40. Rhubarb Chutney with Turkey Cutlets

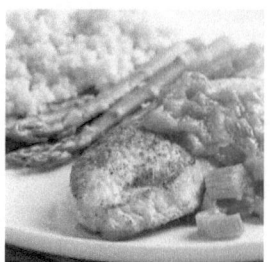

It's time to try rhubarb in this delicious chutney with fresh ginger and golden raisins, served with turkey. You may also pair the sauce with lean pork chops and grilled skinless, boneless chicken breasts. Serve with steamed asparagus and whole-wheat couscous.

Ingredients

- 1/4 teaspoon salt
- 4 (about 1 pound) turkey cutlets, 1/4 inch thick
- 1/4 teaspoon freshly ground pepper, divided
- 1/4 teaspoon ground ginger or 2 teaspoons minced fresh ginger
- 1 tablespoon cider vinegar
- 1/3 cup light brown sugar
- 1/3 cup golden raisins

- Frozen rhubarb (drained, thawed if frozen) or 2 cups sliced fresh
- 1/3 cup chopped red onion
- 2 teaspoons plus 1 tablespoon canola oil, divided

Method

1. Turn the heat to medium and heat 2 tablespoons canola oil in a saucepan. Add onion and stir. Cook until softened for about 4 minutes. Add raisins, rhubarb, vinegar, brown sugar, and 1/8 teaspoon pepper. Turn heat to medium heat and bring the mixture to boil.

2. Stir occasionally until the rhubarb is softened and breaks down (10 minutes). Remove it from the heat ad cover to keep warm. Sprinkle the turkey on both sides with the remaining 1/8 teaspoon pepper and salt. Turn the heat to medium-high and heat the remaining tablespoon canola oil in a large nonstick skillet. Add the turkey and let it cook until just cooked through or browned, 2-3 minutes per side. Now serve the turkey with chutney.

Tips/Notes

Rhubarb is rich in Vitamin C, a very important ingredient to help support the immune system.

41. Maple-Chili Glazed Pork Medallions

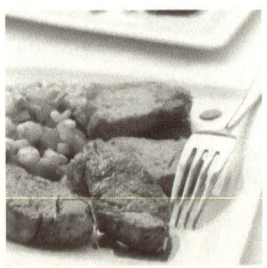

This meal is easy and quick to make and is very tasty when served with a maple-chili glaze in particular.

Ingredients

- 1 teaspoon cider vinegar
- 1 tablespoon maple syrup
- 1/4 cup apple cider
- 2 teaspoons canola oil

- 1-pound pork tenderloin, cut crosswise and trimmed into 1-inch-thick medallions
- 1/8 teaspoon chipotle pepper (ground)
- 1/2 teaspoon salt
- 1 teaspoon chili powder

Method

1. Mix chili powder, ground chipotle and salt in a small bowl, sprinkling over both sides. Turn heat to medium-high and heat oil in large skillet. Add pork and cook until golden, 1-2 minutes per side. Add syrup, vinegar and cider to the pan. Add to boil, scraping up any browned bits.

2. Turn the heat to medium and cook, occasionally turning the pork to coat until the sauce becomes a thick glaze, 1-3 minutes. Serve it drizzled with the glaze.

Tips/Notes

Apple cider is rich in acetic acid which is a great potent antimicrobial and kills most bacteria.

42. Black Bean-Salmon Stir-Fry

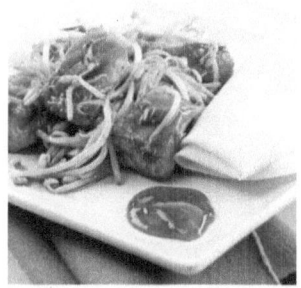

This recipe contains a vitamin C rich bean sprouts and fiber. It's super easy and quick to prepare it and includes rich black bean-garlic sauce and tender salmon cubes. Prepare it and serve with plum sauce and store-bought crepes.

Ingredients

- 1 bunch sliced scallions
- 6 cups mung bean sprouts
- 1-pound salmon, skinned and split into 1-inch cubes

- 1 tablespoon canola oil
- Pinch of crushed red pepper
- 2 teaspoons cornstarch
- 1 tablespoon dry sherry or Shao Hsing rice wine
- 2 tablespoons black bean-garlic sauce
- 2 tablespoons rice vinegar
- 1/4 cup water

Method

1. Whisk cornstarch, crushed red pepper, rice wine or sherry, black bean-garlic sauce and vinegar in a bowl until combined. Turn the heat to medium high and heat the oil in a nonstick skillet. Add salmon and cook for about 3 minutes.

2. Add scallions, bean sprouts and the sauce mixture. Cook, stirring occasionally, until the bean sprouts become tender and cooked down, 2-3 minutes.

Tips/Notes

Health benefits of corn include the control and prevention of diabetes and heart ailments.

43. Sun-Dried Tomato Wraps & Turkey and Corn

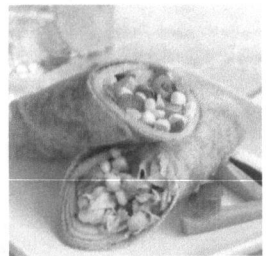

Tomatoes, lettuce and fresh corn kernels make for the most delicious turkey wraps. Add some shredded cheddar or crumbled feta for another layer of flavor. Serve with sliced bell pepper, carrot sticks or crunchy vegetables and your preferred creamy dressing.

Ingredients

- 2 cups chopped romaine lettuce
- 4 8-inch whole-wheat tortillas

- 8 thin slices (about 8 ounces) low-sodium deli turkey
- 1 tablespoon cider vinegar or red-wine vinegar
- 2 tablespoons canola oil
- 1/4 cup chopped soft sun-dried tomatoes
- 1/2 cup chopped fresh tomato
- 1 cup corn kernels, frozen (thawed) or fresh

Method

1. Combine tomato, corn, oil, vinegar and sun-dried tomatoes in a medium bowl. Divide the turkey among tortillas. Top with equal amounts of lettuce and corn salad. Roll up and serve the wraps cut in half (if desired.)

Tips/Notes

Corn provides healthy supportive benefits and contains anthocyanins, the same healthy ingredient found in berries and red wine.

44. Skillet Chicken with Apples & Cranberries

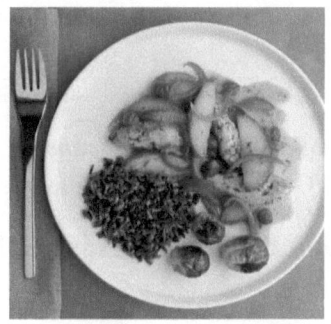

Prepare this delicious meal that comes with chicken cooked in a fast apple-cranberry sauce. In case you enjoy a less part flavor then try the dried cranberries in place of fresh ones. Serve with roasted brussels sprouts and quick-cooking wild rice.

Ingredients

- 1 cup cranberries, frozen (thawed) or fresh
- 1 tablespoon all-purpose flour
- 3/4 cup apple juice or apple cider, divided
- 1 large red onion, sliced and quartered
- 2 crisp red apples, e.g. Braeburn, Gala or Fuji, thinly sliced

- 2 tablespoons canola oil, divided
- 1/4 teaspoon freshly ground pepper
- 3/4 teaspoon salt, divided
- 3/4 teaspoon dried thyme, divided
- 1-pound chicken tenders, trimmed and split into half on the diagonal

Method

1. Sprinkle both sides of chicken with salt, pepper and 1/4 teaspoon thyme. Turn the heat to medium high and heat canola oil in a large skillet. Now turn the heat back to medium and add chicken. Cook and stir until lightly browned on all sides, 3-5minutes total and transfer to a clean plate. Add the remaining tablespoon canola oil to the saucepan. Add onion, apples, the remaining 1/2 tablespoon thyme, salt and 2 tablespoons cider or juice.

2. Stir well to combine and cook until the onion and apples are properly softened, 3-5 minutes. Add the cranberries and sprinkle flour over everything in the saucepan. Cook and stir for about 1 minute. Now place the chicken in the saucepan and add the remaining cider or juice. Cover it and cook, stirring occasionally until the sauce thickens and the chicken is cooked through, about 3-5 more minutes.

Tips/Notes

Cranberries have anti-inflammatory, anti-cancer and antioxidant health benefits. They are also rich in dietary fiber, manganese and vitamin C.

45. Quick Pastrami Hash & Eggs

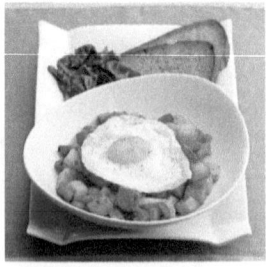

You can always find pre-cooked diced potatoes in the refrigerated section of most supermarkets. This is essential in the preparation of this pastrami hash ultra-fast. (In case you have leftover cooked potatoes, utilize about 3 cups of diced potatoes instead.) Serve this meal with sautéed spinach and rye toast.

Ingredients

- 4 large eggs
- 5 ounces (1 cup) deli pastrami, diced
- 1/4 teaspoon plus a pinch of freshly ground pepper, divided
- 1/4 teaspoon plus a pinch of salt, divided
- 1 teaspoon paprika
- 1 medium green diced bell pepper
- 1 large thinly sliced onion, quartered
- 1 16-18-ounce precooked potatoes, diced
- 2 tablespoons extra-virgin olive oil

Method

1. Turn the heat to medium high heat and heat olive oil in a skillet. Turn the heat to medium and add onion, potatoes, paprika, bell pepper, ¼ teaspoon salt and pepper each. Mix to combine and spread in an even layer in the saucepan. Cook for 3-5 minutes. Add pastrami and spread the back into an even layer and cook undisturbed again until a crust begins to form at the bottom, about 3-5 minutes. Now remove it from heat and cover to keep warm. As soon as you add pastrami to the hash, coat a large nonstick skillet with the cooking spray and place it over medium heat.

2. Crack the eggs into a small bowl and slip them, one after the other, into the skillet. Take care not to break the yolks. Season it with the remaining pepper and salt and turn the heat to medium-low. Cover and cook for about 3 minutes for soft-set yolks. Now divide the hash among the 4 plates and top each serving with an egg.

Tips/Notes

One egg provides just about 75 calories but about 7 grams of high quality protein.

46. Black Bean-Smothered Sweet Potatoes

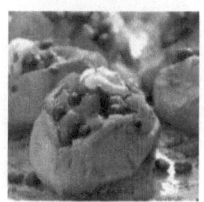

This recipe is easy to prepare and is very satisfying. The fragrant filling of tomato and beans add proteins and vitamins making it nutritionally complete. Remember to consume the potato skin as its full of fiber.

Ingredients

- 2 tablespoons chopped fresh cilantro
- 2 tablespoons reduced-fat sour cream
- 1/4 teaspoon salt
- 1/2 teaspoon ground coriander
- 1/2 teaspoon ground cumin
- 2 teaspoons olive oil
- 1 medium diced tomato
- 1 15-ounce can rinsed black beans
- 2 medium sweet potatoes

Method

1. Using a fork, prick the sweet potatoes. Microwave them on high heat for 15 minutes or until tender. Alternatively, put in a dish and bake until tender (at 425°F). Meanwhile, combine tomato, oil, beans, coriander, cumin and salt in a medium microwave safe bowl. Microwave on high heat for about 3 minutes. You may alternatively heat in a small pan over medium heat. Wait until it gets cool enough to and slash the potatoes lengthwise. Press them open to well the center and add the bean mixture. Now top each one of them with a sprinkle of cilantro and a dollop of sour cream.

Tips/Notes

Cumin comes with several health benefits including its ability to improve immunity, digestion, treating insomnia, asthma, bronchitis, respiratory disorders and piles.

47. Port Sauce & Seared Steak with Pan-Roasted Grape

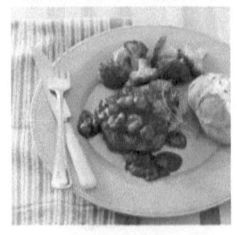

This low-calorie recipe features a quick pan-seared steak with grape sauce and savory-sweet port wine which makes for an incredibly delicious weeknight dinner.

Ingredients

- 1 teaspoon chopped fresh thyme
- 1/4 cup reduced-sodium beef broth
- 1/4 cup port wine
- 1 1/2 teaspoons all-purpose flour
- 1/4 cup diced shallot
- 1 cup seedless red grapes
- 1 tablespoon olive oil plus 1 teaspoon, divided
- 1/4 teaspoon freshly ground pepper
- 1/2 teaspoon kosher salt, divided
- 1/4 pounds boneless strip steak, trimmed

Method

1. Pat the steaks dry and split them into 4 equal portions. Drizzle with pepper and 1/4 teaspoon salt. Turn the heat to medium high heat and heat 1 tablespoon olive oil in a large skillet. Add the steaks and cook for about 5 minutes or until browned at the bottom. Turn it over and reduce the heat to medium-low. Cook for 5 minutes or to your desired doneness. Remove from the heat and set aside. Cover with foil to keep warm.

2. Heat the remaining tablespoon olive oil in the saucepan over medium low heat. Add grapes stir. Keep pressing down on them using the back of a spoon, until the grapes turn golden brown in spots and broken down, 4-7 minutes. Now add shallot and cook. Stir for 1 minute until fragrant. Drizzle with flour. Keep stirring to coat. Add broth, thyme, port and 1/4 teaspoon salt. Increase the heat to medium-high and cook. Stir and scrape up any browned bits until thickened and reduced. Serve the steaks over 3 tablespoons sauce each.

Tips/Notes

Thyme provides a distinct taste that has turned it into a culinary stable. It's gradually gaining a reputation in the treatment of acne and high blood pressure.

48. Smoky Maple-Mustard Salmon

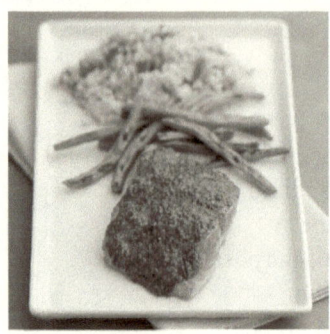

It does not get much delicious –or much easier—than this incredibly speedy recipe for roast salmon with smoky maple mustard sauce. Maple is very sweet and works to balance the tangy mustard; ground chipotle and smoked paprika both add another layer of flavor. Ask at the fish counter to get the salmon split into four 4-ounce fillets with the skin removed. Next, serve it with whole-wheat couscous and roasted green beans tossed with chives and pecans.

Ingredients

- 4 4-ounce skinless center-cut wild-caught salmon fillets
- 1/8 teaspoon salt
- 1/4 teaspoon freshly ground pepper
- 1/4 teaspoon ground chipotle pepper or smoked paprika
- 1 tablespoon pure maple syrup
- 3 tablespoons Dijon mustard or whole-grain

Method

1. Pre-heat the oven to about 450°F. Line a baking sheet with foil and then coat with cooking spray. Combine maple syrup, chipotle or paprika, mustard, pepper as well as salt in a small bowl.

2. Put salmon fillets on the prepared baking sheets. Spread the mustard mixture on the salmon and roast it until just cooked through, 7-10 minutes and serve.

Tips/Notes

Paprika not only adds a spice that adds color to food but is also rich in carotenoids and vitamin C, offering a variety of beauty and healthy benefits.

49. Soba Noodles and Spicy Pork

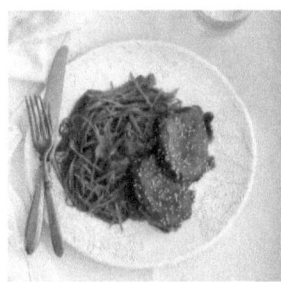

This recipe contains soba noodles which contain less carbs and calories than regular white-flour pasta.

Ingredients

- 2 teaspoons sesame oil
- 2 tablespoons rice vinegar
- 1 red chili pepper chopped and sliced
- 2 sliced scallions
- 1/2 English cucumber
- 1 tablespoon vegetable oil
- black pepper and kosher salt
- 1 1/4-pound pork tenderloin
- 2 ounces soba noodles

Method

1. Cook soba noodles as specified package directions. Season the pork with ¼ teaspoon pepper and ½ teaspoon salt. Heat the vegetable oil in a large skillet over medium-high heat.

2. Brown the pork in batches, 1-2 minutes per slide and transfer it to a larger bowl. Toss it with cucumber, scallions, noodles, sesame oil, vinegar, chili pepper and ½ teaspoon salt.

Tips/Notes

Extremely versatile, you can serve soba noodles hot or cold. They work just well in salads, soups and stir fry's. And because they are made from buckwheat flour, they are great for you. They are also full of iron, amino acids and protein.

50. Black Bean Salad & Zesty Shrimp

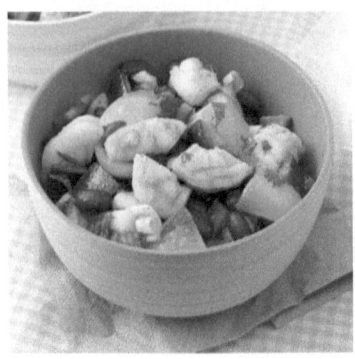

Loaded with peppers, fresh tomatoes and cilantro and seasoned with chile and cumin, this black bean and shrimp salad recipe contains all the flavors of a mouthwatering, fresh salsa. It's also very easy to prepare. Serve with fresh corn tortillas or tortilla chips.

Ingredients

- 1/4 cup chopped fresh cilantro
- 1/4 cup chopped scallions
- 1 large bell pepper or poblano pepper, chopped
- 1 cup quartered cherry tomatoes
- 1 15-ounce can rinsed black beans
- 1 pound deveined and peeled cooked shrimp, split into 1/2-inch pieces
- 1/4 teaspoon salt
- 1 teaspoon ground cumin
- 1 tablespoon minced chipotle chile in adobo
- 3 tablespoons extra-virgin olive oil
- 1/4 cup cider vinegar

Method

1. Whisk oil, vinegar, chipotle, salt and cumin in a bowl. Add beans, tomatoes, poblano or bell pepper, shrimp, cilantro and scallions. Toss to coat and serve cold or room temperature.

Tips/Notes

Some of the greatest health benefits of shrimp include improved brain and bone health, low risk of heart related diseases and weight management.

51. Sicilian Olive Chicken

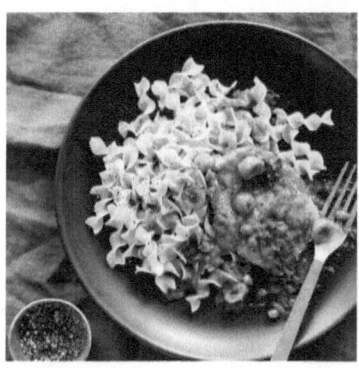

This is a saucy one skillet chicken recipe that includes spinach, olives, tomatoes and capers. You want to try Kalamata olives in place of green Sicilians. Serve over mixed green salad and whole-wheat egg noodles on the side.

Ingredients

- 1 tablespoon olive oil
- 1/4 teaspoon freshly ground pepper
- 4-ounce chicken cutlets
- 1/4 teaspoon crushed red pepper
- 1 tablespoon rinsed capers
- 1/3 cup halved Sicilian or other green olives
- 1 1/2 cups thawed, frozen chopped spinach
- Diced tomatoes with garlic or other Italian-style seasoning

Method

1. Combine spinach, olives, capers, crushed red pepper and tomatoes in a bowl. Drizzle pepper on both sides of chicken. Turn heat to medium heat. Heat olive oil in a large skillet. Cook until browned on both sides, 2-4 minutes. Turn the chicken over and top with tomato mixture. Turn the heat to medium. Cover and cook until just through, 3-5 minutes.

Tips/Notes

Olive oil is rich in phenolic antioxidants and anti-cancer compounds terpenoid ad squalene.

52. Seared Salmon with Green Peppercorn Sauce

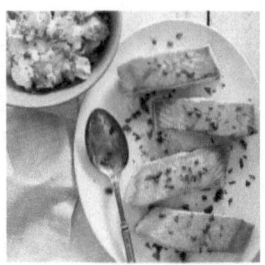

A delicious sauce of butter, lemon juice and piquant green peppercorns top this seared lemon recipe. Green peppercorns are harvested before they mature but come from the same plant as the black ones. When packed in vinegar, they give a pleasantly refreshing sharp flavor. Find them near the capers in most supermarkets. When ready, serve with sautéed kale and red potatoes.

Ingredients

- 1 teaspoon rinsed and crushed green peppercorns in vinegar
- teaspoons unsalted butter, split into small pieces
- 1/4 cup lemon juice
- teaspoons canola oil
- 1/4 teaspoon plus a pinch of salt, divided
- 1 1/4 pounds wild salmon fillet skinned and split into four portions

Method

1. Drizzle 1/4 teaspoon salt on the salmon pieces. Turn the heat to medium high and heat canola oil in a large nonstick skillet. Add the salmon and cook for about 5-7 minutes or until it gets just opaque in the center.

2. Divide and remove from the saucepan from the heat and immediately add peppercorns, butter, lemon juice and the remaining pinch of salt. Swirl the saucepan carefully to seam the butter into the sauce. Top the portions with the sauce.

Tips/Notes

A chemical component in peppercorns known as piperine helps prevent breast cancer from developing. When paired with turmeric, they provide heightened cancer preventing properties.

53. Crab Roll

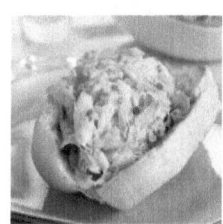

This is a healthier yet low calorie take on a lobster roll that uses crab. It's less expensive but by all means only use lobster if you prefer. Serve with ice-cold beer and coleslaw.

Ingredients

- whole-wheat hot dog buns (toasted, if preferred)
- 8 leaves green or red leaf lettuce
- 12 ounces cooked crabmeat, (preferably drained), any cartilage or shells removed
- 1/4 cup thinly sliced fresh chives, divided
- 1/4 cup finely chopped celery
- 1/4 cup finely chopped shallot
- 1/8 teaspoon salt
- 1/2 teaspoon freshly ground pepper
- 10 dashes hot sauce, e.g. Tabasco
- tablespoons lemon juice
- 1 tbsp. lemon zest, freshly grated
- 1/4 cup low-fat mayonnaise

Method

1. Whisk lemon zest, lemon juice, mayonnaise, pepper, salt and hot sauce in a medium bowl. Mix in celery, shallot and 3 tablespoons chives. Mix well. Gently mix in crab so it does not break too much. Line the buns with lettuce. Now divide the crab filling among the buns and garnish with the remaining tablespoon chives. Serve.

Tips/Notes

Crab is one of the healthiest foods you can ever eat. For a very little amount of calories, you get lots of minerals, protein and a multitude of several B vitamins.

54. Green Beans with Pesto & Poached Cod

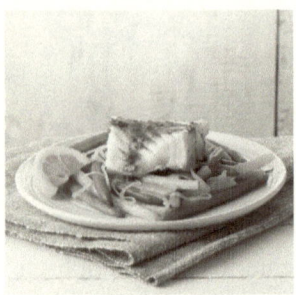

This simple fish recipe uses just one skillet to cook cod right on top of green beans. It uses the same saucepan to prepare a flavorful sauce. The result is a very delicious flaky fish, a savory pan sauce, very tender-crisp vegetables and very little cleanup.

Ingredients

- Lemon wedges for serving
- 1/4 cup prepared pesto
- 1 1/2 cups "no-chicken" broth or low-sodium chicken broth
- 1/4 teaspoon freshly ground pepper
- 1/4 teaspoon salt
- 1 1/4 pounds cod, split into 4 portions
- 3/4 cup thinly sliced shallot
- 1 pound yellow and/or yellow trimmed wax beans
- 1 tablespoon olive oil

Method

1. Turn the heat to medium and heat the olive oil large skillet. Add shallot and beans and stir. Cook until the shallots begin to soften, 1-2 minutes. Drizzle pepper and salt on both sides of cod. Spread beans into a flat layer in the saucepan and lightly place the cod on top. Turn the heat to high. Add broth, stir and cover. Cook until the fish is just cooked through, 4-6minutes.

2. Transfer the cod using a slotted spoon and the beans to a larger serving plate and cover them to keep warm. Turn the heat to high heat and cook the broth until reduced, about 5 minutes. (Do not cover.) Remove from the heat and stir well. Stir in pesto. Pour the sauce over the fish. Serve with lemon wedges. (If desired)

Tips/Notes

Cod provides you protein and B vitamins as well as other several nutrients that help keep your heart healthy.

55. Kale Salad with Preserved Lemon & Walnuts

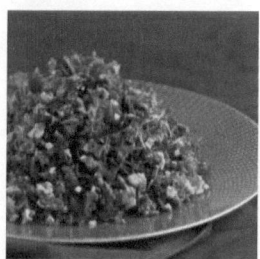

This recipe features kales salad. Massage dressing into the kale leaves until they are coated with flavor and are tender. Topped with the best Mediterranean flavors—walnuts, preserved lemons and olives—this healthy low-calorie salad is incredibly delicious as it is nutritious.

Ingredients

- 2 tablespoons thinly chopped rinsed and preserved lemon rind or rinsed capers
- 1/4 cup pitted quartered Kalamata olives
- 1/2 cup coarsely chopped toasted walnuts
- 10 cups thinly sliced kale
- 1/2 teaspoon freshly ground pepper
- 1 teaspoon dried oregano
- tablespoons lemon juice
- 1/4 cup olive oil
- 1/2 teaspoon salt
- 1 small clove garlic, minced

Method

1. Mash salt and garlic together on a cutting board. Use the side of knife or a spoon to prepare a paste. Transfer it to a larger bowl. Whisk in lemon juice, pepper, oregano and olive oil to combine. Add kale and with clean hands, massage the kale leaves until they are well coated with the dressing for about 1 minute. Transfer the mixture to a platter and sprinkle with preserved lemon or capers, olives and walnuts.

Tips/Notes

Kale is chock full of essential vitamins A, K and C as well as other minerals such as potassium, iron, manganese, copper and phosphorus.

56. Olive Oil & Herb Mashed Potatoes

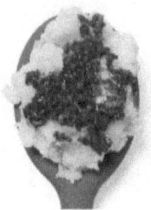

In this healthy low calorie mashed potato recipe, we prepare mashed potatoes with herb-infused virgin olive oil. The green specked mashed potatoes are very delicious and nutritious with chicken or pan-seared pork chops.

Ingredients

- 1 cup buttermilk
- 1/4 cup olive oil
- 1/8 teaspoon white or black pepper
- 1 tablespoon chopped fresh thyme
- 1 tablespoon chopped fresh sage
- 1 tablespoon chopped fresh rosemary
- 1/4 chopped fresh parsley
- 1 clove garlic, minced
- 1 tablespoon salt, plus 1/8 teaspoon, divided
- pounds Yukon Gold potatoes

Method

1. Peel the Yukon Gold potatoes and split then into 2-inch chunks. Place them and 1 tablespoon salt in a large heavy pan. Add cold water to cover by an inch. Bring to boil and turn the heat to a simmer. Cover and cook until the potatoes get very tender, 10-15 minutes. Drain.

2. In the meantime, crush garlic, thyme, sage, rosemary, parsley, 1/8 teaspoon pepper and the remaining 1/8 teaspoon salt in a mortar and pestle until it forms a paste. (Or, finely chop herbs and garlic and combine pepper and salt in a bowl.)

3. Stir in olive oil. Transfer potatoes to a larger bowl and mash with an electric hand-held mixer, a potato masher or by working through a ricer. Stir in the herb mixture, pepper and buttermilk to taste into the mashed potatoes.

Tips/Notes

The health benefits of mashed potatoes include the ability to reduce cholesterol and improve digestion.

57. Salmon Cakes with Olives, Lemon & Dill

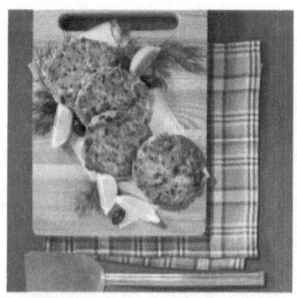

Studded with bright lemon zest, briny olives and a touch of dill, this low calorie, easy salmon recipe is a great one for freezing and for dinner. Whether you serve salmon cakes paired with mixed green salad or on a bun like burger with tomato and lettuce, you want to try lemon juice mixed with a dollop of reduced-fat mayo on top.

Ingredients

- 4 teaspoons olive oil, divided
- 1/2 pounds wild salmon, skinned and split into 2-inch chunks
- 1/2 teaspoon freshly ground pepper
- 1/2 teaspoon salt
- Zest of 2 lemons
- tablespoons coarsely chopped thyme or fresh dill
- 1/2 cup pitted Kalamata olives
- quartered scallions

Method

1. Place olives, thyme or dill and scallions in a food processor. Pulse until finely chopped. Now transfer to a larger bowl. Stir pepper, salt and zest. Pulse the salmon just 3 times to finely chop, not puree. Add

chopped salmon to the bowl and gently mix until mixed well. Alternatively, finely chop scallions, olives, herbs and salmon by hand prior to combining them with salt, pepper and lemon zest.

2. Divide the mixture into 3 separate patties, about 3/4-inch-thick and 3 inches in diameter. Refrigerate before cooking. Turn the heat to medium and heat 2 tablespoons olive oil. Stir in 4 salmon cakes and cook until just cooked through or browned, 8-10 minutes and repeat with the remaining salmon cakes and olive oil.

Tips/Notes

Unlike what most people think, dill doesn't come from a weed. Instead, it's a culinary herb that helps control cholesterol levels and helps relieve the body and mind of insomnia.

58. Three Sisters Succotash

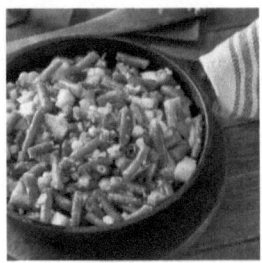

In this pretty easy succotash recipe, beans, squash and corn—known as three sisters—combine as they harmoniously do in the garden. If you are a fan of patty pan squashes, you could use them in place of summer squash or the regular zucchini.

Ingredients

- finely chopped scallions
- 1/4 teaspoon freshly ground pepper
- small zucchini or summer squash, split into 1/2-inch pieces
- 1 tablespoon butter
- 2 tablespoons olive oil
- 2 large ears fresh husked corn
- 3/4 teaspoon salt, divided
- 12 ounces (about 3 cups) green beans, trimmed, split into 3/4-inch pieces

Method

1. Place the beans in a large pan and add water. Add 1/2 teaspoon salt and bring to boil. Cover and turn the heat to maintain a simmer and cook for about 15-20 minutes or until the beans are tender. In the meantime, cut the corns from the cobs and hold an ear by the stem in a deep bowl. Using a sharp knife, chop off the kernels letting them fall into the deep bowl. Scrape down the cob using a small spoon. Do that for the "milk" remaining on the corn pulp and discard the cobs.

2. When the beans are cooked, drain them and reserve the cooking fluid. Heat the butter and oil in a large skillet over medium heat. Add the "milk" and corn and stir to coat. Now stir to coat and add zucchini or squash, beans as well as 2 tablespoons of the bean-cooking liquid. Cook, stirring regularly until the squash and corn are tender, 8-12 minutes. Add more bean-cooking liquid so as to keep the mixture from sticking to the bottom of the pan. Add salt and pepper to season. Sprinkle with the scallions and serve warm.

Tips/Notes

This food contains minimum amounts of saturated fats, cholesterol and sodium. It's an impressive source of thiamin, iron, dietary fiber, potassium, phosphorus, manganese and vitamin C.

59. Turkey Kofta with Tahini Sauce

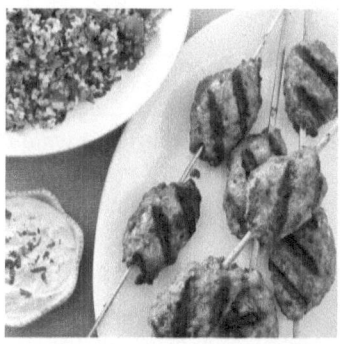

Kofta is a very common term that refers to the act of combining onions, spices and ground meat. In this recipe, minced onion and ground turkey are mixed with allspice and cumin to prepare a delicious grilled dinner. Look for a sesame paste, tahini, with the natural-foods and Middle Eastern Ingredients section of the supermarket.

Ingredients

- 1 tablespoon lemon juice
- 1/3 cup low-fat plain yogurt
- 1/4 teaspoon cayenne pepper
- 1/2 teaspoon salt plus 1/8 teaspoon, divided
- 1/2 teaspoon ground allspice
- 1 teaspoon ground cumin, divided
- 4 tbsp. chopped fresh cilantro
- 1/2 cup dry whole-wheat breadcrumbs or coarse fresh
- 1/2 cup minced onion
- 1 pound 93%-lean ground turkey

Method

1. Preheat grill to medium-high. Pre-heat the grill to medium high. Combine cayenne, turkey, allspice, 1/2 teaspoon salt, 1/2 teaspoon cumin, breadcrumbs, onion and 4 tablespoons cilantro in a large bowl.

2. Gently knead together but avoid overmixing. With clean damp hands, form the mixture into 2 ovals on each skewer and use 1/3 cup for each. Oil the grill rack and grill the kebabs for about 4 minutes per side or until an instant read thermometer inserted in the center registers 165°F. Combine lemon juice, tahini, yogurt and the remaining tablespoon cilantro, 1/8 teaspoon salt, 1/2 teaspoon cumin in a small bowl. Serve the kebabs with the sauce and enjoy.

Tips/Notes

1 tablespoon tahini contains just about 85 calories, 65 of which are made up these essential fats. It also contains several nutrients such as iron, copper, magnesium, phosphorus, manganese and vitamin B_1. It also provides dietary fiber as well as protein.

60. Spiced Salmon with Chili Sauce

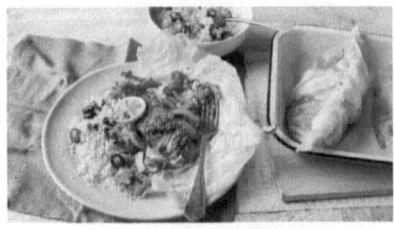

With only 325 calories per serving, this dish is a sure way of enjoying good food while losing weight.

Ingredients (4 servings)

- 4 x 6 ounces salmon fillets
- 2 teaspoon chili sauce
- 1 teaspoon honey
- ¼ teaspoon each of ground red pepper, ground turmeric and salt
- ⅛ teaspoon garlic powder

Method

1. Preheat cooking spray coated broiler. Combine all ingredients except the fish in a bowl and stir with a fork. Rub mixture evenly over fish. Place fillets on broiler, skin-side down. Broil for 8-10 minutes

Did you know?

Chili speeds up the metabolic process therefore it helps you reach your weight loss goal faster?

61. Fish and Baby Tomato Bake

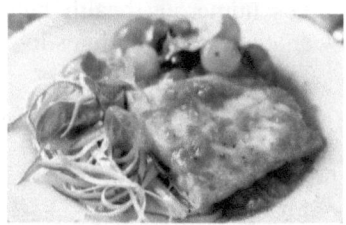

Fish is a healthier substitute for other meat types and has mostly healthy fats and high-quality proteins which both have health advantages for our bodies.

Ingredients (4 servings)

- 4-6 fish cutlets
- 1 tablespoon garlic and herb seasoning
- 4 ounces each of mixed baby tomatoes and steamed Brussels sprouts
- Garlic bulb, halved horizontally
- 3 tablespoons olive oil
- Salt and freshly ground pepper

Method

1. Preheat oven to 200 °C. Grease an oven-proof dish. Season fish with garlic and herb seasoning and place in dish together with tomatoes, garlic and sprouts. Drizzle with olive oil and season with salt and pepper. Bake for 15 minutes. Serve with a salad.

Fun Fact

In Medieval times, garlic was used as a cure for drunkenness and over-eating and in the middle ages, people ate garlic in an attempt to be safe from the Black Death (Bubonic Plague)

62. Pork Kebabs with Chimichurri

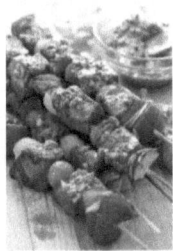

The honey in this dish gives numerous health benefits including boosting immunity, boosting energy and helping with digestion.

Ingredients

- 1½ pounds pork rashers without rind
- 6 peeled and halved baby onions
- 1 tablespoon mustard
- 3 tablespoons honey

For the Chimichurri

- 1 teaspoon each of chopped parsley and dried Italian herbs
- 1 red onion, CHOPPED
- ½ cup olive oil
- 2 tablespoons lemon juice
- 2 garlic cloves, chopped
- ½ teaspoon chili powder
- Salt and freshly ground pepper

Method

1. Preheat oven to 2oo °C. Thread the meat onto kebab skewers alternating with the onions. Mix honey and mustard and use mixture to brush kebabs. Arrange on oven rack and bake for 12-15 minutes. Mix all the chimichurri ingredients while kebabs bake. Serve kebabs with chimichurri and a salad

Mustard Fun Fact

Pope John Paul XXII is believed to have loved mustard so much that he created a new Vatican position of mustard-maker to the pope (grand moutardier du pape) in the early 1300s.

63. Sautéed Minute Steaks

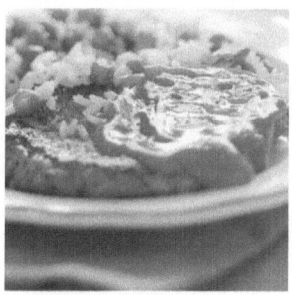

Steak is good for weight loss because it is low in fat and therefore contains less calories. And beef is generally high in protein which is necessary for good health.

Ingredients (serves 4)

- ½ cup flour
- 1 teaspoon garlic salt
- ½ teaspoon pepper
- 20 ounces beef steaks, cubed
- 2/3 cup tomato sauce
- 2 tablespoons each lemon juice and Worcestershire sauce
- 1½ teaspoons ground mustard

Method

1. Thoroughly mix flour, salt and pepper. Use mixture to coat steaks. Grease large skillet and cook steaks over low heat for 4 minutes on

each side. Remove from skillet. Stir in remaining ingredients until heated through. Serve with the steaks

Tips

Tomatoes help keep you focused. They contain anthocyanin, which helps keep memory sharp and also has the potential of positive mood creation.

64. Beef Steak with Mushrooms

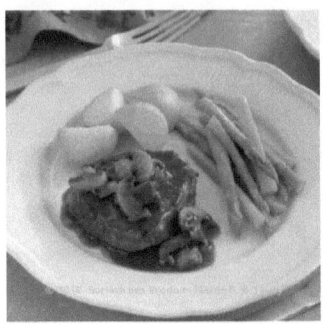

Mushrooms make dishes healthy and are also beneficial for those on weight loss endeavors because they are a low-calorie delicacy because up to 90% of mushrooms is water.

Ingredients

- 1-pound beef rump steak, thinly sliced across the grain into ½cm thick pieces
- 1 cm long chunk fresh ginger, chopped
- 12 ounces spring greens, sliced
- 6 ounces pack sliced mushrooms
- 4 tablespoon oyster sauce
- 2 tablespoon each dark soy sauce and vegetable oil

Method

1. Mix sauces and set aside. Heat a deep skillet until smoking hot, add 1 tsp oil; stir-fry the meat until browned all over. Remove meat and wipe skillet. Add a little more oil. Stir-fry the ginger until golden. Add greens and mushrooms. Stir and cook for 3. Add the steak and soy sauce mixture. Cook for 3 more minutes until sauce thickens a little and everything is thoroughly warmed

Did you know?

Mushrooms are some of the oldest living vegetables and have been used as medicine for thousands of years.

65. Venetian Style Pasta

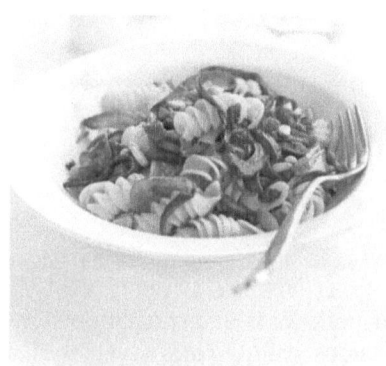

This 20 minute-meal is packed with healthy, low calorie ingredients like raisins and nuts and will ensure loss of weight.

Ingredients (2 servings)

- 2 sliced onions
- 1 tablespoon canola oil
- 8 ounces pasta screws
- 4 teaspoon balsamic vinegar
- 2 tablespoon each raisins and toasted pine nuts
- 5 ounces spinach, chopped

Method

1. Boil pasta for 8-10 minutes. Put oil in pan and fry the onions till slightly brown. Stir in vinegar, raisins, capers and most of the nuts into the onions and cook for 2 minutes. Stir in spinach with a little water. Toss drained pasta with mixture and divide. Scatter remaining nuts into serving dishes.

Did you know?

The variant vitamins and minerals in spinach have skin therapeutic attributes to leave skin healthier and more radiant.

66. Pork Panfry

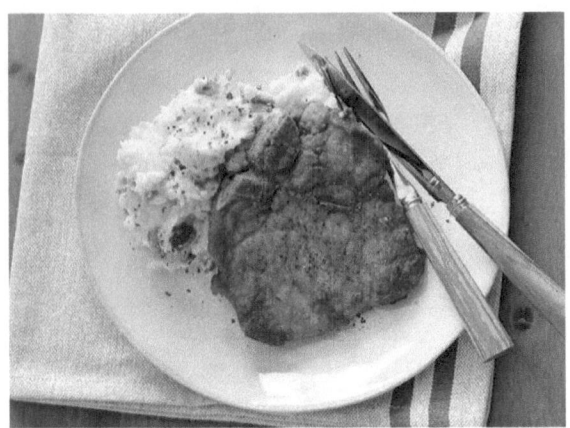

The main ingredients of pork loins and mushrooms ensure that this dish has many health benefits besides weight loss advantages, these include fighting various cancers.

Ingredients

- 18 ounces pork loin fillet
- 1 tablespoon flour
- 2 teaspoon dried rosemary
- 3 tablespoon olive oil
- 9 ounces sliced mushrooms
- Finely chopped garlic clove
- 300 ml vegetable stock

Method

1. Cut pork into finger thick strips. Coat well with a mixture of the rosemary, flour and some salt and pepper. Heat 2 tablespoons of oil in a wide frying pan and fry pork until browned on both sides. Remove from pan. Heat remaining oil and fry mushrooms for 2 minutes. Sprinkle in garlic and return pork to pan. Stir in the stock until mixture boils. Simmer until pork is cooked.

Fun fact

Not only does garlic have many uses from medicinal to flavoring; it is also believed to fight off evil spirits and keep vampires away.

67. Sealed Hake with Olive Salsa

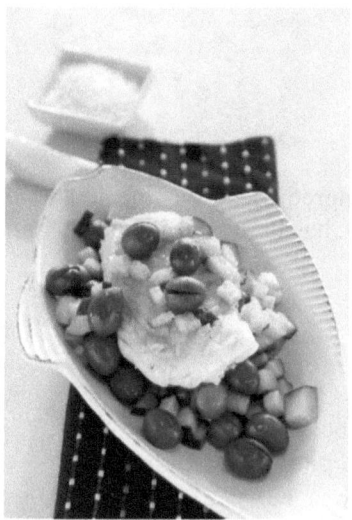

Not only does hake encourage weight loss, it contains Omega 3 fatty acids which have numerous health benefits including improving brain functionality.

Ingredients (serves 4)

- 4 hake fillets
- 2 tablespoons melted margarine
- 1 cup black olives
- 1 cup thinly sliced cucumber
- ¼ cup oil
- 1½ tablespoon vinegar
- Salt and pepper to taste

Method

1. Heat the pan. Meanwhile, brush fillets with melted margarine and season. Fry hake for 7 minutes on each side. Mix olives and cucumber in a bowl, sprinkle with oil and vinegar. Season well and serve with salsa.

Olives Fun Facts

An olive tree is believed to live up to 3000 years and some of the oldest olive trees are believed to be in the Mount of Olives, in Israel.

68. Sweet and Sour Pork

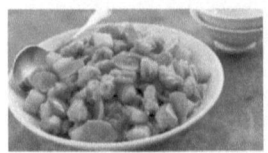

Lean pork is the main ingredient in this meal. This makes the meal good for weight loss because pork has high protein content and a significant number of essential nutrients.

Ingredients

- ¼ cup oil
- 1 tablespoon minced fresh ginger
- 18 ounces cubed pork all fat trimmed
- 1 tablespoon soy sauce
- 2 tablespoons sweet chili sauce
- 1 cup canned pineapple, drained
- 1 cubed red pepper
- 2 sliced spring onions
- Pepper to taste

Method

1. Heat the oil in a pan. Fry ginger for 3 minutes. Add pork and fry for 4 more minutes. Add the rest of the ingredients and cook for 3 minutes. Season well and serve.

Did you know?

Pork is the most versatile meat and can be cooked through stir and pan frying, baking, boiling, barbecuing, grilling, microwaving and roasting among other cooking methods.

69. Broccoli and Cauliflower Primavera

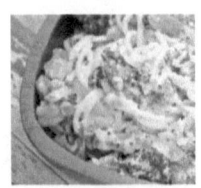

The ingredients in this dish make it one of the dishes with the most weight loss friendly qualities especially because all ingredients are very low calorie and are used in most fast weight loss diets.

Ingredients

- ¼ cup vegetable oil
- 1-pound cauliflower florets
- 1-pound broccoli florets
- 1 pound sliced carrots
- 18 ounces screws pasta
- ½ cup grated parmesan cheese

Method

1. Boil the pasta according to package instructions and drain. In a frying pan, heat the oil and add vegetables. Season with salt and pepper. Fry for 4 minutes ensuring you don't overcook. Add the pasta and mix well. Sprinkle with cheese and serve.

Did you know?

Cabbage and broccoli help in cancer prevention. They are both cruciferous vegetable and this family of vegetables is linked to significant reduction in risk of cancer, especially ovarian cancer, prostate cancer, breast cancer, colon cancer and bladder cancer.

70. Bacon Wraps

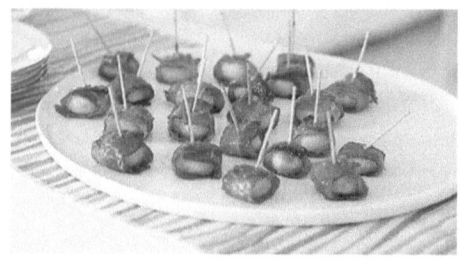

Ingredients (8 servings)

- ½ cup margarine
- 3 cups chopped rind-less bacon
- 3 cups sliced leeks

- 8 wraps
- Pepper for seasoning

Method

1. Melt the margarine in a frying pan and fry bacon for 8 minutes. Add leeks and cook covered for 3 minutes then add seasoning. Spoon equal amounts of mixture on wraps' centers and fold wrap from bottom, ensuring you cover only half the mixture. Fold from the sides to form a wrap. Roll and serve.

Leeks Fun Fact

The Welsh of old believed in the power on the leeks which they put in their helmets when going to war, believing that leeks would ensure they were victorious.

71. Beef and Broccoli Stir-Fry

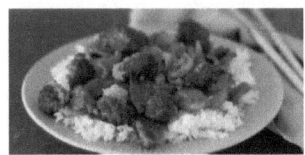

Enjoy this delicious meal without spending lots of time to prepare. With only 430 calories, losing weight is guaranteed.

Ingredients

- 8 ounces sirloin steak
- 1 teaspoon cornstarch
- 2 tablespoon cooking oil
- 1 thinly sliced onion
- 3 minced garlic cloves
- 1 tablespoon minced ginger
- 4 cups chopped broccoli

For the sauce

- $^2/_3$ cup chicken stock
- ¼ cup hoisin sauce
- 2 tablespoon oyster sauce
- 2 tablespoons soy sauce

- 4 tablespoons cornstarch
- 1 tablespoon rice vinegar
- 1 teaspoon sesame oil
- ½ teaspoon chili paste

Method

1. Prepare sauce by whisking together all the sauce ingredients. Set aside. Cut beef into thin strips across the grain and toss with cornstarch. Heat 1 tablespoon oil in deep skillet over high heat. Stir fry beef for 3 minutes and put in separate bowl. Add remaining oil to skillet and stir-fry onion, garlic and ginger for a minute. Add broccoli and ½ cup water and steam for 3 minutes. Pour in sauce and stir for until sauce thickens. Stir in beef and any juices for 3 minutes.

Did you know?

Broccoli has all beneficial components found in vegetables, one of which, indole-3-carbinol is known to prevent hormone related cancers like prostate and breast cancers.

72. Roast Sea Bass with Orange and Honey

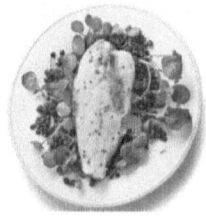

It takes 20 minutes to make this dish which is not only tasty and low calorie but also gluten free for those allergic to gluten

Ingredients

- 2 large sea-bass fillets
- Zest and juice ½ orange
- 2 teaspoon each honey and mustard
- 2 tablespoon olive oil
- 9 ounces ready-to-eat lentils
- 3 ounces watercress
- Small bunch each parsley and dill, chopped

Method

1. Heat oven to 200°C. Place fillets skin-down on individual foils. Mix honey, zest, mustard, ½ oil and some seasoning; drizzle mixture over fillets. Pull foil sides up and twist edges. Place foils on baking tray and bake for 10-12 minutes. Warm lentils and mix with remaining ingredients. Divide into 2 plates, place fish on top and drizzle any left juices and serve.

Fun fact

A third of male fish in British waters is undergoing sex change due to pollution in human sewage.

73. Broiled Tilapia Parmesan

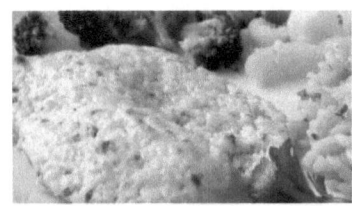

Tilapia is the main ingredient in this dish and it helps you lose weight because it has no carbohydrates, no sugar and very little fat and therefore very little calorie count.

Ingredients

- ¼ cup parmesan cheese
- 2 tablespoons each of butter and mayonnaise
- 1 tablespoon lemon juice
- ⅛ teaspoon each of dried basil, celery salt, onion powder and ground black pepper
- 1-pound tilapia fillets

Method

1. Preheat broiler and spray no-stick spray. Mix all ingredients except fish in a bowl. Single layer the fillets on pan and broil a few inches from heat for 3 minutes. Flip and redo. Remove from oven and put cheese mixture on top side. Broil until topping is browned and fish flakes easily.

Did you know?

Tilapia can help you maintain a healthy blood pressure while keeping many diseases at bay because it is a good source of Omega 3 fatty acids.

74. Teriyaki Fried Rice with Chicken

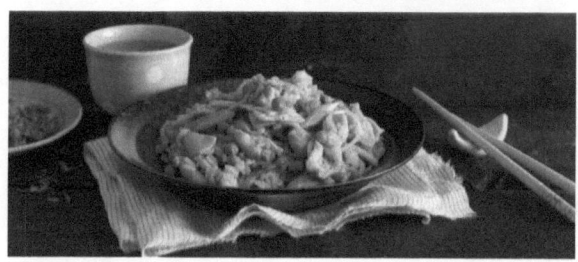

Chicken is good for weight loss because unlike beef and pork, it is low in fat but high in protein and therefore low in calories.

Ingredients (4 servings)

- 5 ounces chicken breasts
- 1½ tablespoon vegetable oil
- 2 onions, chopped
- Small carrot, julienned
- Small beaten egg
- 2½ cups cold cooked rice
- 2 tablespoons Kikkoman Roasted Garlic Teriyaki Marinade and Sauce
- 1 teaspoon chili paste
- 1 tablespoon soy sauce

Method

1. Cut chicken into thin strips. Heat oil in large skillet over high heat. Put chicken, onions, carrot and chili sauce and stir-fry until chicken is cooked. Add egg and stir gently until firm and stir in rice and cook until heated through. Add Teriyaki sauce and soy sauce and remove from heat and mix well.

Fun fact

Chickens can't taste sweetness in foods but can detect salt and most choose to avoid it.

75. Spicy Beans and Rice

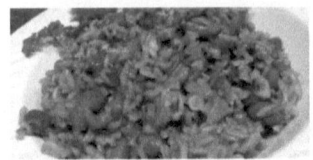

This dish is rich in spices and spices are known for greatly aiding weight loss. Spices are known to speed up metabolism which in turn helps you lose weight faster.

Ingredients (4 servings)

- 2 tablespoon canola oil
- 1 chopped onion
- 1 chopped chili
- ½ tablespoon minced fresh ginger
- ½ tablespoon ground turmeric
- 1½ tablespoons ground cumin
- 2 cups cooked red beans
- 4 cups cooked white rice
- Salt and pepper

Method

1. Heat oil in a frying pan. Add and fry the onions until soft. Add the remaining ingredients except rice and cook for ten minutes. Add rice and cook until heated through. Season and serve.

Did you know?

Beans contain folate which is essential for brain health because it helps by reducing the levels homocysteine, an amino acid which can reduce brain function.

76. Onion and Cheese Tarts

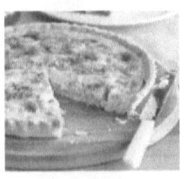

Every ingredient in this dish is nutrient packed and that makes the dish highly nutritious. The dish is low in calories and carbs and contains many health benefits from the nutritious ingredients.

Ingredients

- 1 pastry roll
- ¼ cup Dijon mustard
- 1 large onion, sliced
- 1 cup grated cheddar cheese
- 1 sliced tomato
- 1 teaspoon vegetable oil
- Salt and pepper

Method

1. Preheat oven to 200⁰C. Heat oil in a pan and slightly fry the onions. Lightly flour a pastry board and place the pastry on top. Cut pastry into small squares and spread mustard. Spoon fried onion, sprinkle with cheese and top with a tomato slice. Place on greased baking tray and bake for 10 minutes.

Did you know?

You do your teeth great service by eating cheese, cheese has a very high content of calcium, which you need for strong teeth.

77. Tomato Tartlets

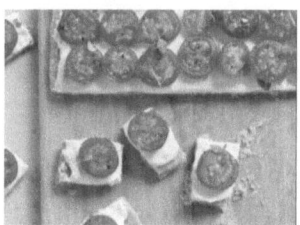

This dish is easy, fast and healthy to allow the enjoyment of tasty food while losing weight and saving time.

Ingredients (serves 5)

- 1 roll puff pastry
- ½ cup basil pesto

- 2 large tomatoes, sliced
- 5 cheddar cheese slices
- Basil leaves to serve

Method

1. Preheat oven to 200 °C. Roll out pastry onto lightly floured surface and cut into 2cmx2cm squares. Cut cheese slices into same size as pastry squares. Spread pesto onto the pastry and arrange the tomatoes and cheese slices on top. Cover with another pastry square. Bake until golden brown and serve with basil.

Fun fact

Limburger cheese and humans share a common bacterium which causes the cheese's unpleasant odor and unpleasant human odor.

78. Curried Broccoli and Cabbage

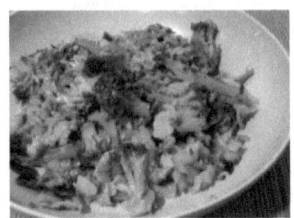

The power of this dish lies in the many spices which, besides giving it variant flavors which you will enjoy, aid in faster weight loss through speeding up metabolism.

Ingredients (8 servings)

- 4 tablespoons oil
- 1 chopped onion
- 1 fresh ginger, chopped
- 1 teaspoon ground turmeric
- 2 tablespoons curry powder
- 2 green chilies, chopped
- 1 cup canned tomato
- 1 large cabbage, shredded
- 2 cups each broccoli florets and chopped carrots
- Handful chopped coriander

Method

1. Heat the oil in a frying pan. Add and fry onions until soft. Add all the remaining ingredients except coriander. Reduce heat and cook covered for 10 minutes. Add coriander just before serving.

Did you know?

Cabbage and broccoli help in cancer prevention. They are both cruciferous vegetable and this family of vegetables is linked to significant reduction in risk of cancer, especially ovarian cancer, prostate cancer, breast cancer, colon cancer and bladder cancer.

79. Mushroom and Cabbage Stroganoff

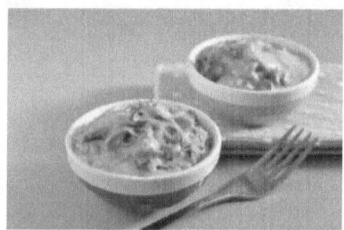

This dish has the potential to aid in weight loss. The protein it provides from the mushrooms keeps you full for a long time and prevents hunger pangs.

Ingredients (8 servings)

- 4 tablespoons oil
- 1 large onion, chopped
- 2 tablespoons paprika
- 4 pounds sliced mushrooms
- 1 white and 1 red cabbages, shredded
- 3½ cups vegetable stock
- 1-pound double cream
- Salt and pepper

Method

1. Heat oil in a large frying pan. Add onions and fry until soft. Add paprika, cabbage and mushrooms and cook for 3 minutes. Add stock and simmer covered, for 8 minutes. Add the cream and season well then cook for a further 4 minutes before serving.

Did you know?

Cabbage is a cruciferous vegetable a type of vegetables linked to significant reduction in risk of variant cancers. In addition, cabbage can stop running tummies and improve appetite.

80. Summer Cabbage Soup with Sausages

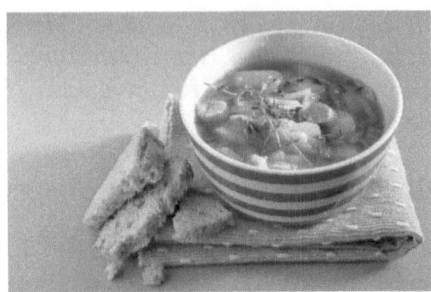

The sausage and cabbage combination in this dish makes the dish highly feeling and ensures loss of weight through keeping you full for longer.

Ingredients (serves 8)

- 4 tablespoons oil
- 1 chopped onion
- 1 sprig thyme
- 8 ounces pork sausages, cooked and sliced
- 1 cabbage, shredded
- 4 medium potatoes, cubed
- 6 cups vegetable stock
- Pepper to taste

Method

1. Heat the oil in a saucepan. Fry the onions in oil until soft. Add the remaining ingredients. Cover and cook for 10-15 minutes. Season well and serve.

Did you know?

Potatoes contain nutrients like vitamin C, B and potassium which are good for relieving inflammation of the intestines and the digestive system. Potatoes are soft; are easy to digest therefore are good for those with mouth ulcers.

81. North African Cabbage

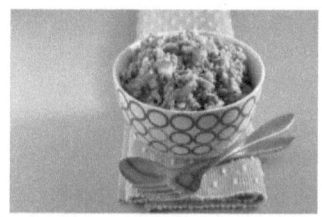

This is one of the lowest calorie foods you can ever enjoy and with this dish; losing weight is a sure thing. The peppers in the dish also help with increasing the metabolic rate.

Ingredients (5 servings)

- ¼ cup oil
- 1 white cabbage, shredded
- 1 tablespoon each of garam masala and cumin
- ½ deseeded green pepper, thinly sliced
- Salt and pepper

Method

1. Heat the oil in a frying pan. Add cabbage and stir fry for 3 minutes. Add everything else but green pepper and stir fry for another 3 minutes. Add green pepper and fry for another 3 minutes. Serve with couscous.

Did you know?

The cabbage family of vegetables is linked to significant reduction in risk of cancer, especially ovarian cancer, prostate cancer, breast cancer, colon cancer and bladder cancer.

82. Cheese Crumpets

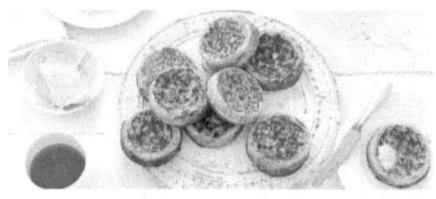

This dish is a highly filling dish because of the crumpets and sausages and will therefore help in weight loss through keeping away the hunger pangs.

Ingredients (6 servings)

- 6 crumpets
- ½ cup Dijon mustard
- 2 cups, cooked and sliced pork sausages
- 1 thinly sliced onion
- 2 cups grated cheddar cheese

Method

1. Preheat oven to 220°C. Place the crumpets on a baking tray. Spread mustard on each crumpet and bake until cheese melts. Serve immediately.

Did you know?

Crumpets are a slightly sweet bread snack alike to flapjacks and can be enjoyed sweet or savory.

83. Four Bean Salad

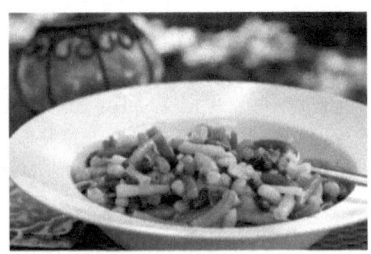

This salad is filling and this makes you keep your weight under wraps because you will not get hunger pangs. In addition, beans are very nutritious and are a high-level protein food.

Ingredients (serves 6)

- 3 cups blanched green beans
- 2 cups cooked speckled red beans
- 2 ½ cups cooked white beans
- 2 each of green peppers medium onions, sliced
- 1 cup each white vinegar and olive oil

- 3 tablespoons caster sugar
- ½ cup chopped fresh coriander
- Salt and pepper

Method

1. Place beans, peppers and onions into a salad bowl and mix gently. Put the remaining ingredients into a jug and whisk briskly to make the salad dressing. Sprinkle salad dressing over salad and immediately serve.

Coriander Fun Fact

The ancient Egyptians believed that coriander could be used in the afterlife as food for the dead, whom they believed were living another life.

84. Singed Steak, Tomato and Blue Cheese Salad

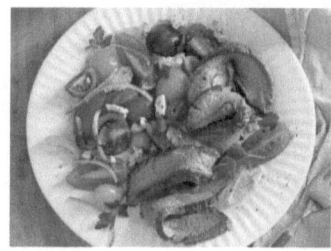

This dish has the benefits of protein from the beef, the high protein value in beef can keep you full for longer and can help keep hunger pangs at bay.

Ingredients (serves 4)

- 1 pound trimmed steak
- 4 teaspoons olive oil
- ¾ teaspoon kosher salt
- ¼ cup each of crushed blue cheese and finely chopped red onion
- 1½ teaspoons white wine vinegar
- 20 ounces quartered grape tomatoes

Method

1. Brush steak with 1 teaspoon olive oil and sprinkle with ¼ teaspoon pepper and ½ teaspoon salt. Heat a large skillet over high heat until almost smoking. Add steak to pan and cook each side for 2½ minutes.

Place on cutting board and cool for a few minutes before cutting into thin slices, across the grain.

2. Combine all remaining ingredients except cheese, onion and tomatoes, and stir briskly. Add tomatoes, onion and steak to mixture and toss. Divide mixture into four plates and sprinkle the cheese evenly.

Did you know?

Eating cheese in moderation helps prevent tooth decay and protects enamel like most tooth pastes.

85. Potato, Bacon and Avocado Salad

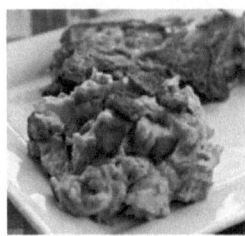

This salad in one of the healthiest foods you can eat while chasing a weight loss plan, the low-calorie ingredients in this dish contain some of the healthiest benefits in one ingredient.

Ingredients (8 servings)

- 6 large potatoes, cubed
- 1-pound bacon bits, fried
- 3 tablespoons each of chopped parsley and olive oil
- Salt and pepper
- 2 cubed and peeled avocados

Method

1. Place potatoes, bacon, parsley and olive oil in a bowl. Season and mix well. Add avocados, toss lightly and serve.

Did you know?

Avocados are considered among the healthiest foods on the planet because they contain more than 25 essential nutrients and up to 15 health benefits.

86. Mexican Salad

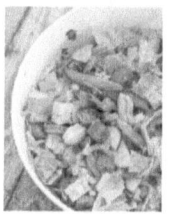

This dish is very healthy because it has avocados which are considered among the healthiest foods on the planet; containing more than 25 essential nutrients and up to 15 health benefits.

Ingredients (serves 8)

- 4 tablespoon oil
- 3 tablespoon lemon juice
- 1 tablespoon Mexican spice
- 1 large iceberg lettuce, shredded
- 3 large tomatoes, cut into wedges
- 3 cups tinned kidney beans, drained
- 2 avocados, sliced
- 2 thinly sliced red onions

Method

1. Whisk the oil, lemon juice and spice in a bowl. Mix all salad ingredients in a salad bowl. Sprinkle the oil mixture over the salad and serve.

Variety Tip

For a meaty option, fry ground/ minced meat with the Mexican spices

87. Garlic Chicken with Egg Plant Salad

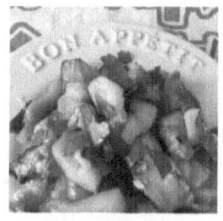

This recipe, with its Mediterranean touch, will excite your taste buds and your belly. Made with very basic ingredients, this recipe has excellent nutritional value for those looking to lose weight.

Ingredients

- ½ pound chicken breasts
- 1 Medium sized Eggplant
- 1 tbsp. soy sauce
- ½ tsp of ginger and garlic paste
- Salt and pepper to taste
- Chopped Parsley for garnishing
- Extra virgin olive oil

Method

1. Brush your chicken fillets and sliced eggplant with soy sauce and let them rest. Add salt, pepper and ginger garlic paste to the chicken fillets and leave the chicken to marinate for about 15 minutes. Preheat the oven to medium heat. Toss the marinated chicken and eggplant into the over and sprinkle olive on top. Let it cook for about 20 minutes before you take it out and serve. Garnish with parsley and if you want, you can add a tinge of lemon juice for the aroma.

Three Reasons Why Eggplants Are Good for You

One cup of eggplant has only twenty calories, so it is excellent for those looking to eat and not gain weight. Not only does scientific researches prove that eggplant is an excellent agent to reduce weight, it is said to reduce the risk of heart diseases and diabetes. It also promotes healthy complexion and hair, increase energy and lose weight overall.

88. Cod Served with Corn, Beans and Pesto

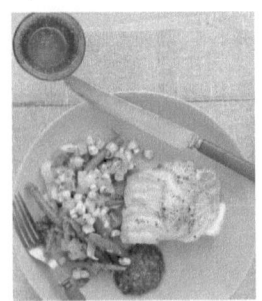

Tossing a little store-bought pesto to the corn and bean salad is an excellent innovative treat to your taste buds

Ingredients

- ½ Pound Cod
- ¼ cup corns
- ¼ cup beans of your choice
- A handful of store bought pesto
- Salt and pepper to taste
- Olive oil

Method

1. In a lightly greased skillet lay the cod and season it with salt and pepper. Let the cod cook for two minutes on each side and then plate. Toss the corns, beans and pesto in a bowl with salt pepper and some olive oil. Serve the cod with your corn, bean and pesto salad.

Three Reasons Why Red Beans Are a Healthy Alternative

One cup of red beans fulfills 58% of your daily requirements for folate. They are excellent source of dietary fibers. They are considered part of two food groups; the vegetable and the protein group, which makes them great for weight loss.

89. Walnut, Beets and Goat Cheese Salad

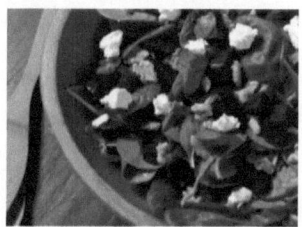

After a long day at work, this is what you need! Made with a handful of walnuts, it is a unique assortment of goat cheese and beets for the food connoisseurs.

Ingredients

- A handful of walnuts
- Steamed beets

- ¼ cup goat cheese cubed
- Salt and pepper to taste
- ½ tbsp. Orange juice

Method

1. Toss in the walnut, beets and goat cheese in a bowl. Season with salt pepper. Just before you serve, add orange juice.

Three Reasons to Incorporate Goat Cheese into Your Diet

It is easier on the human digestive system and low in calories. It is not implicated to result in heart diseases. Also, it is a good source of calcium, protein, vitamin A, vitamin K, phosphorus, niacin and thiamin.

90. Steak Salad with Mango Cubes

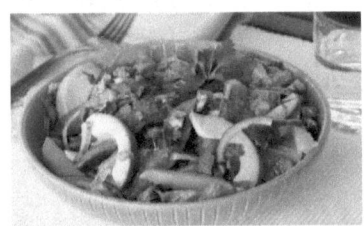

This Asian recipe with a twist is guaranteed to add variety and color to your table and your life! The tinge of honey accentuates the roasted beef and mango combination.

Ingredients

- Roasted beef slices cubed
- A tinge of honey
- A tinge of lemon
- A pinch of grated ginger
- ½ tsp of soy sauce
- Mango-peeled and cubed

Method

1. Roast beef with ginger and garlic in the oven till it's done. Now, use the roasted beef and toss it in with ginger, soy sauce and mango. Right before serving, add honey and lemon.

Benefits of Honey

Honey is one of the best anti-bacterial agents. It is proven to help prevent cancer and heart diseases. Regular use of honey increased athletic performance.

91. Spinach and Garlic Vinaigrette

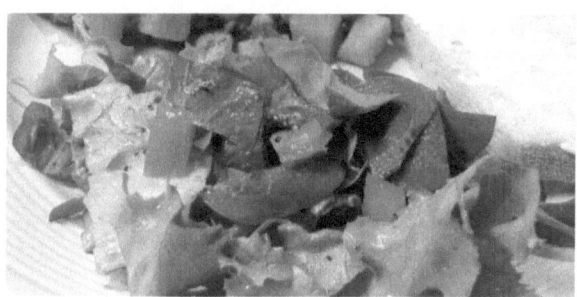

Assort this simple recipe with your favorite main course and use it instead of bread or rice to cut down on your calories This savory combination will make you love spinach.

Ingredients

- 6 ounces of blanched baby spinach
- Grated garlic clove
- A sprinkle of olive oil
- Black pepper and salt to taste
- ¼ cup vertically sliced red onion
- ¼ tsp Dijon mustard
- 1 tbsp. of white vinegar

Method

1. Combine the garlic, mustard, vinegar, salt pepper and olive oil to make your dressing. Coat it over the spinach and onion salad right before serving. Garnish with some oregano flakes, if you want (optional).

Health Facts About Spinach

Excellent source for dietary fiber. Ideal source for vitamin-K and calcium. Helps in muscle build-up and reduce fat deposit.

92. Quinoa served with Mushrooms, Kale, and Sweet Potatoes

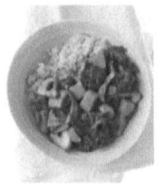

An excellent vegetarian alternative for meat lovers, filled with nutritional value and taste. Sweet potatoes and kale add the uniqueness, taste and color to this wondrous delight!

Ingredients

- 1 cup quinoa, boiled
- Olive oil as needed
- ½ cup peeled, boiled and cubed sweet potatoes
- 10 ounces of your favorite mushroom, sliced
- 1 bunch kale, stems discarded and blanched
- 2 cloves grated garlic
- ½ cup dry white wine
- Grated parmesan to garnish

Method

1. In a saucepan, golden brown mushrooms and cubed sweet potatoes with a little olive oil. Stir in the garlic. Add kale and the rest of the ingredients till the vegetables are soft. Serve with quinoa and sprinkle parmesan.

Three Reasons Why You Should Incorporate Kale in Your Diet

Kale has zero fat. Kale is high in iron. Also, it is an excellent detox food.

93. Pea Risotto with Baked Spinach

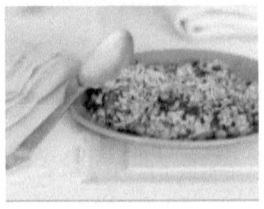

An easy fix after a long day, this recipe requires no stirring and bakes in the oven until creamy and ready to be served.

Ingredients

- 1 tbsp. unsalted butter
- 1 chopped shallot
- Black pepper and salt to taste
- 1 cup Arborio rice
- 1 cup frozen peas
- 3 ounces of baby spinach, chopped
- Parmesan for topping
- 3 cups of broth of your choice (vegetable or chicken)

Method

1. Preheat the oven at 400 degrees. Take an oven-proof dish, add all the ingredients and bring them to boil. Toss the dish into the oven for 25 minutes or until the rice is creamy. Top it off with some parmesan and you are good to go!

Why Incorporate Garlic in Your Diet?

Garlic-rich diets help control weight. Garlic is low in calories and very rich in vitamin C. It can combat sickness, including the common cold and help you stay healthy.

94. Braised Chicken with Radish and Baby Carrots

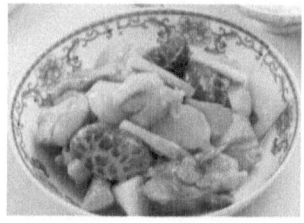

This beautiful golden chicken recipe is an excellent dinner recipe served with fresh radishes and baby carrots

Ingredients

- 8 pieces chicken thighs, boned-in
- Olive oil for cooking

- 1 cup chicken broth
- 12 medium radishes - diced
- ¾ pound of Baby carrots
- 1 tsp sugar
- Salt and pepper to taste
- 2 tbsp. chopped chives

Method

1. Season the chicken with salt and pepper. Place the chicken thighs in a heated Dutch oven and cook for 6 minutes on each side, then plate. With the broth, add in radishes, carrots and sugar in the Dutch oven. Place the chicken on top of the vegetables and let it simmer on low heat, partly covered for 15 minutes. Garnish with chives.

Three Reasons Why Radish Is So Good for You

Radishes are good for your stomach and your liver. Radishes are very filling and excellent for weight loss. They are good appetizers and act as mouth and breath fresheners.

95. Pumpkin Soup

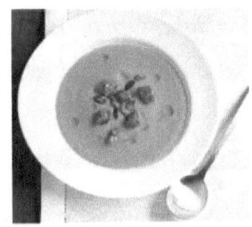

With an enticing color, this recipe is good to look at and good to eat! With few ingredients, this recipe is packed with nutrition and taste for a large family dinner.

Ingredients

- 1 chopped onion
- 2 slices chopped bacon/beef (if you prefer)
- 29-ounce canned pumpkin
- 3 ½ cup chicken broth
- 1 cup applesauce
- ½ cup sour cream

98. Cumin Chicken on a Bed of Black Beans

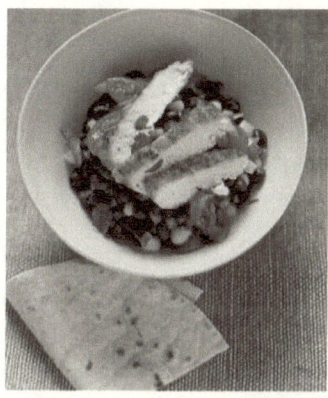

Packed with health, this is a superb mix of vegetables and seasoned chicken breasts for your appetite

Ingredients

- 2 chicken breasts, sliced
- 1 tsp ground cumin
- Salt and pepper to taste
- 1 jalapeno pepper
- 3 cups canned black beans
- 1 cup corn kernels
- 2 tbsp. red wine vinegar
- Cilantro for garnishing

Method

1. Rub the chicken breasts with cumin, black pepper and salt. Let it marinate. Heat oil and sauté the chicken 4 minutes on each side and transfer it to a cutting board. Add the rest of the ingredients (except for cilantro and vinegar) in the pan you just sautéed chicken in and toss the ingredients for a couple of minutes, then add vinegar. Assort in a plate and place the sliced chicken on top. Garnish with cilantro.

Benefits of Black Beans

Packed with protein and fiber, black beans move through the digestive track slowly, making you feel fuller. Its use can decrease your chances of cardiovascular diseases. It is also an excellent anti-oxidant.

99. Meatball Soup with Escarole

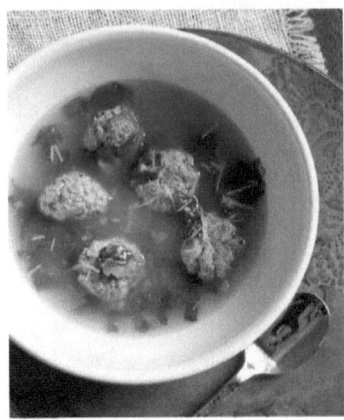

A scrumptious recipe of meat and vegetables, this soup will serve six and be an excellent companion on a nice supper table

Ingredients

- ½ pound lean ground beef
- 6 tbsp. of grated parmesan cheese
- 6 tbsp. of plain bread crumbs
- ¼ cup parsley
- 2 eggs lightly beaten
- 2 chopped onions
- 8 cups of escarole, shredded
- 2 diced carrots
- 14 ounces of chicken broth
- Salt and pepper to taste

Method

1. Toss in meat, eggs, half of the parmesan, bread crumbs, salt and pepper into a chopper and make meatballs from the blended mixture. In a skillet, with a tablespoon of olive oil, cook meatballs until browned, then plate. With one tablespoon of oil, add the rest of the ingredients and let the broth cook for 15 minutes.

2. Add escaroles and simmer for another five minutes. Add meatballs and bring the broth to boil. Let it simmer for another five minutes. Serve with grated parmesan cheese.

Escaroles are Great for You. Why?

Best source for vitamin K as per USDA's agricultural research. High in vitamin C, which enables healthy glowing skin and nails. Very low in calories and excellent weight reducing agent.

100. Chickpea Salad with Red Chili Flakes

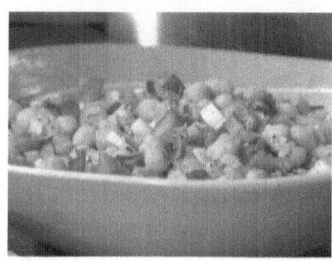

This traditional subcontinental delight has been used as a weight controlling snack since long. The unique texture of the chickpea, combined with red chili flakes, makes it a perfect quick fix.

Ingredients

- 1 can chickpeas, drained and rinsed
- Red chili flakes to your taste
- Salt to taste
- Coriander leaves to garnish
- ½ onion, diced
- 1 tomato, diced
- 1 green chili, finely chopped
- ½ tsp Lemon juice
- A pinch of Chat Masala

Method

1. Take a bowl and toss in all the ingredients. Garnish with coriander leaves. You are done!

Chickpea for Weight Loss

Chickpea are packed with fiber which stimulates weight loss. It helps you stay full, longer. It belongs to the legume family and like all legumes; it is highly advised to those looking to shed some extra pounds but can't resist food!

101. Sautéed Mushroom and Chicken Sandwiched in a Bran Bread

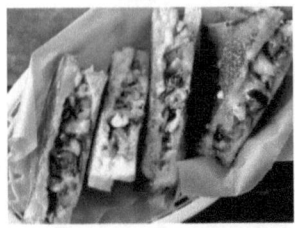

A perfect snack for the day out, this easy recipe is made with chicken breast and golden browned button mushrooms.

Ingredients

- 1 piece Chicken breast
- Salt and pepper to taste
- 1 tbsp. Soy Sauce
- A pinch of garlic powder
- 2 slices Bran bread, grilled/toasted
- 1 tbsp. Yogurt
- ½ tsp tomato ketchup
- 3 diced Mushrooms

Method

1. Marinate chicken with salt, pepper, soy sauce and garlic powder. In a skillet, with very little olive oil, sauté chicken for 5 minutes on both sides, then transfer to a plate.

2. In the same skillets add the chopped mushrooms and sauté until they go golden brown, then plate them with the chicken. Mix together yogurt, tomato ketchup with a dash of salt and pepper for the spread. Take the grilled/ toasted slices of bran bread and spread the yogurt mixture. Place the chicken and mushroom on the bran bread spread with yogurt sauce. Add some sliced tomatoes and onions if you want and gobble away!

Bran Bread and Health Benefits

Reduces the risk of metabolic syndrome. Proven to reduce the risk of Type 2 Diabetes substantially. Helps prevent gallstones.

102. Grilled Chicken Thighs on a Bed of Brown Rice

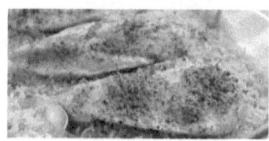

An excellent alternative to deep fried chicken, this recipe offers taste and health, all together! Paprika and cumin together give this recipe a very unique taste.

Ingredients

- 2 chicken thighs, boned-in
- ½ tsp paprika powder
- A pinch of cayenne
- Salt and pepper to taste
- ½ cup beer
- Olive Oil for grilling
- 1 cup cooked brown rice

Method

1. Use all the ingredients and marinate the chicken. Refrigerate the marinade for two hours. It's better to use a zip lock bag, toss in the marinade before you let it rest for two hours. Grill the chicken pieces in a preheated oven at 400 degrees for around 30 minutes. Alternately, you can also bar-b-q the chicken for some smoked flavor. Serve with brown rice.

Paprika Health Benefits

It helps lighten skin and improve complexion. It has some great anti-aging qualities, ladies! It also prevents hair loss and helps maintain hair color.

103. Egg and Rocket Pizza

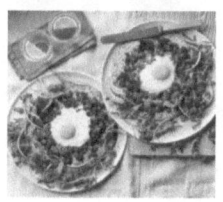

This is a new recipe made with tortillas instead of the traditional pizza bread. Break an egg on top of the tortilla and toss it in the oven. You have made your own hearty egg and rocket pizza with a modern twist.

Ingredients

- 1 tortilla bread
- 1 egg
- Tomato puree
- 1 tbsp. chopped parsley and dill
- Olive oil for brushing the tortilla bread
- 20-30 grams pack rocket
- Salt and pepper to taste
- ½ onion, diced

Method

1. Preheat the oven and 200C. Lay the tortillas on two baking sheets and brush olive oil. Bake the tortilla brushed with olive oil in the oven for 3 minutes. Spread the tomato puree, salt and pepper over the tortilla bread you took out of the oven. Break an egg in the center of the tortilla and bake the bread for another 10 minutes in the oven. Serve scattered with rocket. Add onions if you want and you are done!

Eggs for Your Health

Egg white is very low in calories and it is recommended that you consume egg white for your dose of calcium and protein. Eggs are filling and cheap, they will let you stay healthy inside a budget. Using eggs can also prove to be very healthy for your physical appearance because of its high protein value.

104. Oats with Fruits and Nuts Topped with Greek Yogurt

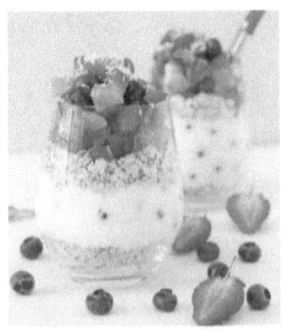

Made with Porridge oats, this recipe uses low fat Greek yogurt to make a perfectly healthy breakfast/evening snack. Oranges and nuts add to the aroma and texture of the recipe

Ingredients

- 6 tbsp. porridge
- 2 oranges
- 100 ml of low fat Greek yogurt
- An assortment of nuts, berries and seeds

Method

1. Cook oats in 400 ml of water. Let the oats simmer until a paste is formed. Cut oranges into pieces after removing the pith of the oranges. Pour the porridge into a bowl, serve with low fat Greek yogurt and an assortment of orange pieces, nuts, berries and seeds. A number of variations of this recipe can be made with the fruits and nuts of your choice!

Use Yogurt

Yogurt is an excellent low-fat alternative to cream. It helps you feel light and active. With low-fat yogurt in the market, you can enjoy it all you want without fearing any calorie. Yogurt is also good for your skin.

105. Thai Prawn Fried Rice

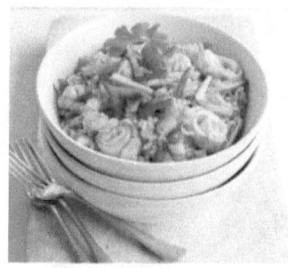

A mouth-watering Asian recipe that is prepared in a total of 25 minutes. Made with prawns, this recipe comes with a unique combination of eggs and rice.

Ingredients

- 800 grams of rice, cooked. Use leftovers, if any
- 300 grams of peeled prawns

- 2 tbsp. red Thai curry paste
- 2 tbsp. vegetable oil
- 2 lightly beaten eggs
- 100 grams of green beans
- 1tbsp. Thai fish sauce
- Sliced green chili and coriander leaves to garnish

Method

1. Heat oil in a wok. Pour in the eggs and let then eggs cook. Do not stir. Let it form an omelet at the bottom of the pan. Cook for about 1 minute, till the omelet is set. Tip the omelet out onto a chopping board, roll it up and slice it into ribbons. Set aside.

2. Heat the curry paste in the wok with a tablespoon of water. Toss in the rice to coat them with the curry paste. Add the prawns and let it heat through. Add in the rest of the ingredients and toss. Plate it out with egg strips, green chili and coriander leaves- chopped and set aside for garnish.

Shrimp on A Diet!

High in protein, it adds variety to the table. It is simple and easy to cook and packed with vitamins. With one serving, you will consume half of your daily requirement of selenium for the day along with other nutrients, which is why it is advised to be part of your diet at least once a week.

106. Baked Sea Bass with Lemon and Capers

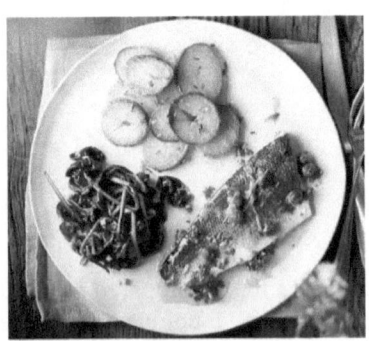

This nutritious gluten free recipe will take you on a joy ride of taste and color. Made with sea bass, this simple recipe is an ideal for quick fix dinners. The capers add nutrition and color to the golden, baked sea bass.

Ingredients

- 100-gram sea bass fillet
- 1 tbsp. of olive oil
- Lemon zest
- 1 tbsp. small capers
- 1 tsp. gluten free Dijon mustard
- 2 tbsp. parsley

Method

1. Make the caper dressing first by adding lemon zest, mustard, capers and seasoning in a pinch of water. Heat the baking oven at 220C and line the baking tray with baking parchment. Now, on the baking parchment, place the sea bass, skin side up. Rub in some salt and olive oil. Bake the fish for around 7 minutes and then plate with a spoonful of dressing on top. Sprinkle with parsley.

The Goodness of Capers

Capers have extraordinary antioxidant powers. It is packed with minerals, such as iron, calcium and copper. It helps destroy byproducts in in meat that are rich in fat, which makes it a healthy choice to be paired with meat.

107. Confetti Pesto Pasta with Diced Chicken and Green Beans

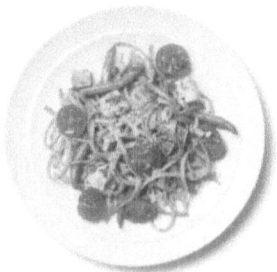

This parting recipe is easy and delicious. Made with chicken, this is another recipe for connoisseurs of good food who are also health conscious!

Ingredients

- 1/3 cup diced chicken breasts
- ¼ cup pesto sauce
- ¼ pint cherry tomato

- 1/3 cup cooked green beans
- Salt and pepper to taste
- 1 cup cooked linguine
- Parmesan for topping

Method

1. Toss in all the ingredients together in a bowl other than the linguine. Do not add parmesan as well, we are leaving it for the end. Right before serving; add the sauce you just prepared over a plate on linguine and garnish with parmesan. Enjoy!

Green Beans and Health Benefits

With excellent levels of vitamin A, green beans are great for your eyes. They are also rich in vitamin C. So next time you meet somebody with great skin, they might just be eating a lot of beans! Did you know that green beans are very low in calories and contain NO saturated fat?

108. Steak and Pepper Tacos

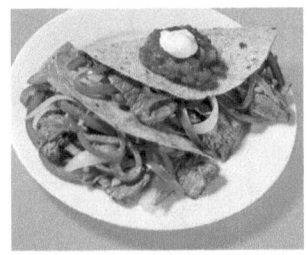

A completely healthy meal that fulfills your requirement of proteins without compromising your diet plan, 'Steak and pepper tacos' is a very easy to cook recipe which does not take too much of your time. Served with jalapenos, corn and avocado, this dish is a perfect blend of meat and vegetables.

Ingredients

- One pound of flank steak
- Juice of one lime
- One teaspoon kosher salt
- Two crushed garlic cloves
- Half teaspoon chili powder
- Three teaspoons vegetable oil

- Half sliced red onion
- Three thinly sliced bell peppers
- Half cup corn kernels
- Eight warmed corn tortillas
- Half sliced avocado
- Quarter cup Monterey Jack
- Quarter cup salsa Verde
- Two tablespoons jalapenos (sliced and pickled)

Method

1. Marinate the steak on lime juice, salt, garlic and chili powder and let it rest for some time. Take a pan and add two teaspoons vegetable oil in it and heat it for five minutes. Put the red onion, bell peppers and corn in the pan and heat the vegetables while tossing. When the peppers turn brown, stop heating them and transfer them into a plate. Now add another teaspoon of oil in the pan and lay the marinated steak in it.

2. Cook the steak at medium high temperature for about eight minutes and turn it a couple of times. Slice the cooked steak if required and serve it with peppers and onions and use tortillas, salsa Verde, jalapenos and avocado if required.

Did you know?

Flank steak is cut from the abdomen of a cow and can be used as an alternative to skirt steak which is a major ingredient of fajitas.

109. Shrimp and Avocado Rice Bowl

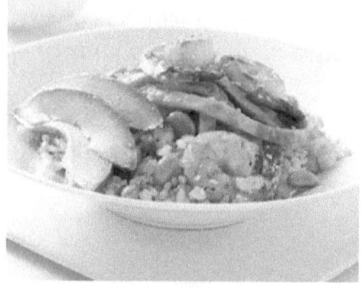

A tasty rice and meat dish, shrimp and avocado bowl lets you enjoy a complete seafood meal as sesame seeds, brown rice and delicious shrimp make a mouth-watering combination.

Ingredients

- Sixteen medium tail-on shrimps
- Two teaspoons sesame oil
- One and a half teaspoons honey
- Some cayenne peppers
- Two lightly beaten eggs
- One tablespoon soy sauce
- One tablespoon vinegar
- Two teaspoons sesame seeds (toasted)
- One and a quarter cup short-grain cooked brown rice
- One sliced ripe avocado

Method

1. Cook the shrimp in a medium high heated pan after adding sesame oil, honey and a pinch of cayenne pepper. Turn the shrimp a couple of times and cook it for two minutes per side. Take another pan and after adding some more sesame oil in it, introduce the eggs. Let them stand for a couple of minutes and when they are set, turn them. When the eggs are ready, put them on a chopping board and slice them into several pieces.

2. Take some soya sauce, vinegar and honey in a bowl and mix them. Add the sesame seeds to the rice and top it with the shrimp, avocado and eggs strips. Put the soya sauce vinegar mixture on the table and use it to add to the taste.

Did you know?

Shrimp contain high levels of omega-3 which is a very important component of a healthy diet. They also have negligible amounts of mercury which is harmful and can cause cancer.

110. Lemon Walnut Chicken

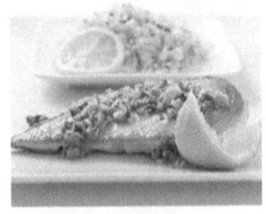

Lemon is a major constituent of 'Lemon Walnut Chicken', and is incredibly good for health. The chicken used in this recipe is cooked in olive oil which is also a low-cholesterol type of edible oil.

Ingredients

- Two tablespoons chopped parsley
- Two tablespoons chopped and toasted walnuts
- Quarter teaspoon grated lemon zest
- Four medium skinless and boneless chicken breast pieces
- Two teaspoons flour
- Half teaspoon salt
- Half teaspoon black pepper
- One tablespoon extra-virgin olive oil
- Three tablespoons diced shallots
- Quarter cup low-sodium chicken broth
- One tablespoon fresh lemon juice
- One and a quarter cup brown and steamed basmati rice

Method

1. Mix the chopped parsley, walnuts and lemon zest in a bowl and let it stand for some time. Take some chicken broth and sprinkle some flour, salt and black pepper on it. Now, warm a large pan and add in it, the shallots. Heat the shallots until their color changes. Add the chicken breast pieces in the pan and heat them until their color changes to brown. Now pour the broth and lemon in the pan and heat the contents even further until the liquid thickens.

2. Take the chicken pieces out and add the parsley and lemon zest sauce in the pan. Mix the ingredients of the pan and pour the sauce on top of the cooked chicken. Serve the chicken with the steamed basmati rice and use lemons for dressing.

Did you know?

Basmati rice is a type of long grain rice which is cultivated in Pakistan and India and is a major export of both countries.

111. Spinach Mushroom Pizza

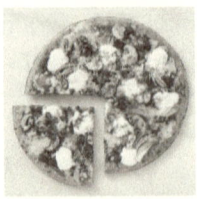

A vegetable pizza is a kind of dish not many of us have heard of, but the Spinach Mushroom Pizza is a one of a kind. Containing spinach, mushrooms and mozzarella, this dish really does the word 'Pizza' justice.

Ingredients

- One 12-ounce wheat pizza crust
- Quarter cup pizza sauce
- Half cup thawed and drained frozen spinach
- A quarter of small thinly sliced red onion
- One cup shredded mozzarella
- Six medium sliced mushrooms
- Quarter cup ricotta
- Two tablespoons grated Parmesan
- One tablespoon extra-virgin olive oil
- Two teaspoons balsamic vinegar

Method

1. Preheat the oven to medium high and put a baking sheet in it. Place the pizza crust on a surface and put some sauce, spinach and onion on it. Dust the crust with the mozzarella and mushrooms and add ricotta while spraying olive oil all over.

2. Use a cutting board to transfer the pizza to the preheated baking leaf in the oven. Bake the crust for ten minutes until it is inflated and beginning to turn brown at the edges and has melted cheese on the top. Take the ingredients out and preheat the broiler. Heat the pizza until the cheese is browned and sparkling. Let pizza cool on the sheet for some time. Add some balsamic vinegar, cut into pieces, and serve.

Did you know?

Spinach is abundant in iron and calcium in addition to Vitamin K, Vitamin C, Vitamin A, magnesium and manganese. These nutrients are vital in the proper functioning and growth of a human body.

112. Chickpea Tagine

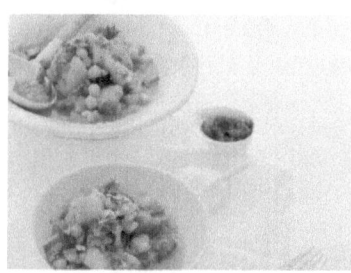

Chickpea Tagine is an amazing meat-free dish that is rich in nutrients and contains cumin, garlic, almonds, chickpeas, zucchini and apricots in perfect amounts.

Ingredients

- One and a half tablespoon extra-virgin olive oil
- One quartered and sliced red onion
- Half teaspoon salt
- Two sliced small carrots
- One and a half cup butternut squash (cubed and peeled)
- Two chopped garlic cloves
- Three peeled pieces of fresh ginger
- Two teaspoons honey
- One teaspoon ground cumin
- One whole cinnamon stick
- Quarter teaspoon turmeric
- Four cored and chopped plum tomatoes
- One quartered and cut medium zucchini
- Ten sliced dried apricots
- Half cup water
- One 19-ounce drained and rinsed can of chickpeas
- Freshly squeezed juice of half a lemon
- One cup whole wheat couscous
- Four teaspoons almonds (sliced and toasted)

Method

1. Add olive oil in a large pan and add onions and salt and cook and stir for five minutes. Add the sliced carrots and heat for five more minutes. Add butternut squash, ginger and garlic and raise the heat while stirring. Introduce some honey, cinnamon stick, cumin and

turmeric and mix for one minute. Add the tomatoes, apricots and zucchini and stir well. Pour some water and heat to the boiling point. Cover the pan and reduce the heat as needed to boil while mixing from time to time, until the vegetables are soft.

2. Add the chickpeas and lemon juice and raise the heat until the chickpeas are cooked enough and the liquid has thickened. Season the dish with additional salt, honey, and lemon. Garnish with sliced almonds and serve.

Did you know?

Almonds are a rich source of oils that are low in cholesterol and carry great nutritional value.

113. Penne with Broccoli and Ricotta

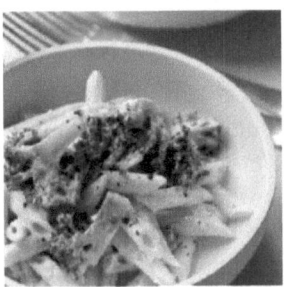

If you are finding something that is easy to cook and does not take much time, Penne with Broccoli and Ricotta is your answer. This recipe contains good quantities of ricotta, garlic, turkey sausages and broccoli and is a perfectly balanced diet.

Ingredients

- A small amount of salt
- One bunch of broccoli
- Twelve ounces whole wheat penne
- One tablespoon extra-virgin olive oil
- Two lean Italian turkey sausages without casings
- Half sliced medium red onion
- One sliced garlic clove
- A small amount of crushed red pepper flakes
- Two tablespoons tomato paste

- Quarter cup part-skim ricotta
- Two tablespoons grated Parmesan

Method

1. Take a pan of salted water to the oven, add the broccoli and cook the pan for some four minutes. Take the broccoli to a sieve and after cooling it for some time, chop it into medium sized pieces. Add the wheat penne to the same pan of boiling water and heat. Reserve half a cup of the pasta in the hot water before draining the penne.

2. Meanwhile, medium heat the olive oil and add the sausages, garlic, onion and red pepper flakes and cook while turning the sausages with a wooden spoon until they get browned. Add the chopped broccoli until tender and heat for two more minutes. Introduce the tomato paste and cook while mixing, until a balanced mixture is obtained.

3. Lower down the temperature of the oven and add the pasta to the mixture. Toss to homogenize the contents and add some of the hot water to wet the ingredients if they seem dry. Mix the ricotta and Parmesan and take the pan out of the oven while tossing thoroughly. Serve immediately.

Did you know?

Parmesan is a type of pale colored cheese which has its roots in Parma, an Italian city. It is used as a seasoning for dishes like Pizza, Lasagna and Spaghetti.

114. Cumin Salmon with Yogurt-Cucumber Sauce

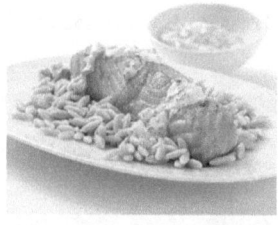

This Salmon dish which is served with a delicious (and good for health) yogurt-cucumber sauce and a blend of delicious raw vegetables is an amazing option when you are looking to satisfy your hunger without putting in too much effort.

Ingredients

- Two teaspoons extra-virgin olive oil
- Half teaspoon ground cumin
- Half teaspoon sugar
- Half teaspoon black pepper
- Half teaspoon salt
- Four salmon fillets
- Half cup non-fat Greek yogurt
- One large peeled, seeded and diced pickling cucumber
- One trimmed and finely chopped scallion
- Three tablespoons minced fresh parsley
- One teaspoon fresh lemon juice
- Eight ounces whole wheat orzo

Method

1. Take the olive oil, sugar, cumin, black pepper, and half a teaspoon of salt in a bowl. Put the salmon on a baking leaf and sprinkle the top with the oil mixture. Allow the salmon to stand and refrigerate it for around twenty minutes. Preheat the oven to a medium high temperature range and mix the yogurt, scallion, cucumber, parsley, lemon juice, and the rest of the salt in a small bowl. Heat the fish for around ten minute and dress with the yogurt sauce and serve immediately.

Did you know?

Salmon is one of the most farmed edible fish in the world and contributes about $10 billion to the US economy every year.

115. Hearty Roast Beef Panini

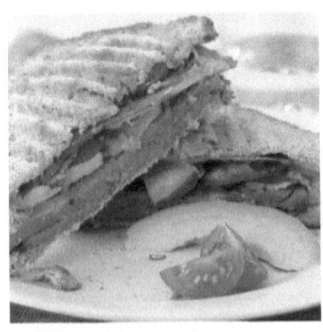

Beef is normally considered a high calorie food – not anymore. The low-fat bread and roasted lean beef used in this recipe do nothing to harm your diet and the tomato slices and avocado improves the flavor of the dish twofold.

Ingredients

- Two slices of low-fat multigrain bread
- Two ounces deli-sliced, store-roasted, lean beef
- Two beefsteak tomato slices
- Quarter sliced avocado
- Quarter cup baby arugula
- One teaspoon Dijon mustard
- Quarter teaspoon extra-virgin olive oil

Method

1. Put a slice of bread in a plate and cover it with the roasted beef, avocado slices, tomato slices and arugula. Spread some mustard on the other piece of bread and combine some mustard with arugula. Put a nonstick pan on the stove and heat it at a medium low temperature. Brush some oil on the sides of the bread and put it in the pan. Put a heavy steel plate or pan on top of the piece of bread and heat it until it gets brown and slightly warm. Serve it with some fresh salad.

Did you know?

Dijon mustard was invented in 1856 when the acidic syrup of young grapes was replaced by vinegar in the typical mustard recipe.

116. Turkey Meatloaf with Walnuts and Sage

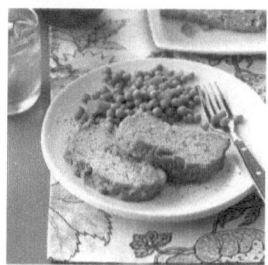

This recipe is made from a list of healthy ingredients which include wheat bread, fat-free milk, walnuts and Parmesan cheese, and parsley, carrots and garlic enhance the taste of turkey breast even more.

Ingredients

- Two teaspoons olive oil
- One large grated carrot
- Four sliced scallions
- One minced clove garlic
- Half a cup of walnuts
- Two slices of whole wheat bread
- Quarter cup fat-free milk
- Two lightly beaten egg whites
- One-pound lean turkey breast
- Quarter cup chopped fresh parsley
- Quarter cup grated Parmesan cheese
- One teaspoon dried sage
- Half teaspoon salt
- Half teaspoon freshly ground black pepper

Method

1. Heat the oven up to about 350°F, stick a foil to baking sheet and spray some olive oil on the foil. Put some oil in a pan and heat it at a medium high temperature range. Add the scallions, carrot, and garlic and cook for three minutes with constant stirring.

2. Wait for the vegetables to get tender and remove them from the oven. Meanwhile, introduce the walnuts into a food processor and chop them down using a metal blade. Break the pieces of bread down and add them in the processor to mix them homogenously with the walnuts. Put the crumbs in a bowl and mix milk and egg white in them.

3. Add the parsley, turkey, cheese, salt, sage, pepper, and the mixture prepared in the previous step. Mix the contents thoroughly until they blend perfectly. Shape the mixture into a loaf and bake for about an hour and let it stand for some time before slicing it into pieces as required.

Did you know?

Walnuts are a healthy source of proteins and also contain dietary fiber and many essential amino acids as well.

117. Slow Cooker Moroccan Chicken with Olives

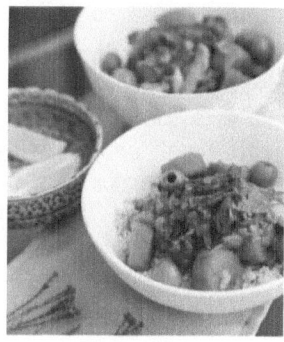

If you are looking to put your dinner on the stove to be cooked and rest while it does, Moroccan chicken with olives is the perfect recipe for you. This dish contains a delicious combination of coriander, cilantro, black olives, tomatoes and cooked chicken breast.

Ingredients

- Half cup chicken broth
- Quarter cup all-purpose flour
- Three tablespoons olive oil
- Two teaspoons ground cumin
- Half teaspoon freshly ground black pepper
- Quarter teaspoon salt
- One can stewed tomatoes
- One sliced carrot
- One large onion
- Thirty small pitted black olives
- Three minced cloves of garlic
- Two pounds of chicken breast (boneless and skinless)
- Half cup chopped fresh cilantro
- Three quarters cup of dried red chili peppers
- One teaspoon ground coriander
- One teaspoon ground caraway seed

Method

1. Cover the slow cooker with cooking spray and add the flour, broth, oil, pepper, cumin, and salt in it and mix the contents until smooth. Add the carrot, tomatoes, olives, onion and garlic and stir to mixture. Put the chicken in the cooker and cover it with the other ingredients

while heating at a high for three to four hours or at a low for five to six hours.

2. Clean the peppers by removing the stems and seeds from them and throwing them away. Dip the peppers in water for about an hour until they soften. Put them in a food processor with a metallic blade and add the coriander, garlic, salt and caraway seed. Pulse the contents until a paste is formed. Sprinkle some oil in the food processor so that consistency is achieved. Also add the cilantro in the processor and mix thoroughly. Garnish the dish as desired and serve immediately.

Did you know?

Even though coriander possesses a lime like flavor and is used widely for preparing a number of recipes all around the world, it can cause an allergic reaction in some people.

118. Chicken Piccata

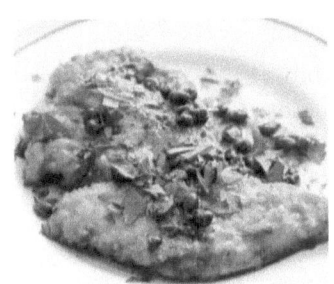

Fans of simple, easy to cook dishes won't find many better options than Chicken Piccata, which is a tasty combo of chicken tenders, lemon juice and parsley. This recipe features some good herbal ingredients as well in addition to the protein rich constituents.

Ingredients

- Twelve ounces of chicken tenders (boneless and skinless)
- Two tablespoons flour
- Four tablespoons olive oil
- Freshly squeezed lemon juice
- Two tablespoons chopped fresh parsley
- Two teaspoons minced capers
- Freshly ground black pepper

Method

1. Put the chicken tenders on a chopping board and flatten it by using a rolling pin. Put the tenders in the flour. Heat a large pan at a medium high temperature and add some oil in it until it starts sizzling. Put the chicken in the pan and cook it, turning each piece every two minutes.

2. Take it out when the chicken becomes brown and crispy. Add some parsley, lemon juice and capers and boil the mixture. Reduce the temperature and allow it to stand so that the flavors blend in perfectly. Season the chicken as required and serve.

Did you know?

Capers are a common component of the Maltese and Italian cuisines and are used predominantly as a garnish.

119. Slow Cooker African Chicken Stew

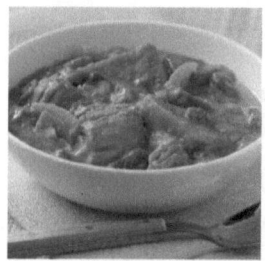

One of the most famous and delicious African dishes, the African Chicken Stew has high nutritional value due to the ingredients like peanut oil, chicken thighs, sweet potato and peanut butter, and even though, it takes some time to get cooked, the recipe is well worth the wait.

Ingredients

- One tablespoon peanut oil
- Twelve ounces of chicken thighs (boneless and skinless)
- One chopped onion
- Three minced cloves of garlic
- One chopped and seeded jalapeno chili pepper
- One thickly sliced carrot
- One peeled and cubed sweet potato
- One can of chicken broth
- Half cup of unsalted peanut butter

- Two tablespoons tomato paste
- Quarter teaspoon salt
- Quarter teaspoon freshly ground black pepper

Method

1. Heat a large sized pan to medium high temperature and add some oil in it. Add chicken in the pan and cook the contents with constant stirring until the meat turns brown. Transfer the contents to a slow cooker. Take the pan back to the stove and add onion, chili, garlic, carrot and pepper. Cook the vegetables for a minute and transfer them to the cooker as well. Stir in the sweet potato, peanut butter, tomato paste and broth to add to the taste.

2. Cook the contents of the cooker on a high temperature for three to four hours or on a low temperature for five to six hours until the ingredients become tender. Garnish the stew with carrot slices, garlic and sweet potato and add salt and black pepper as required.

Did you know?

Although peanut butter is rich in nutrition, it can be very harmful for people suffering from a peanut allergy, and can even cause death if such a reaction is not treated immediately.

120. Spicy Olive and Turkey Pita Sandwich

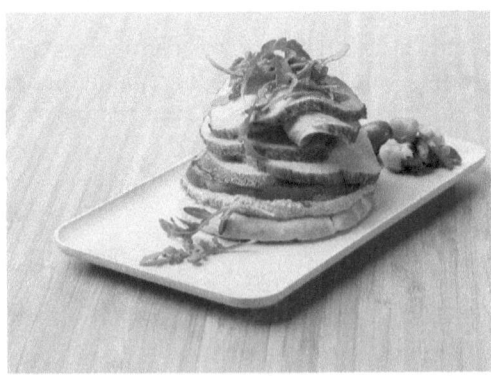

This dish contains a combination of green and black olives which are used for dressing the turkey breast patty that is used for making this amazing sandwich. Wheat pita bread is used in this recipe in addition to a small amount of mixed greens and red pepper flakes.

Ingredients

- Ten pitted and chopped green olives
- Ten pitted and chopped black olives
- One teaspoon balsamic vinegar
- One teaspoon extra-virgin olive oil
- Quarter teaspoon red-pepper flakes
- 1 whole halved wheat pita
- Four ounces deli-sliced turkey breast
- Half cup mixed greens

Method

1. Combine the green olives, vinegar, black olives and red-pepper flakes in a small bowl. Fill two ounces of turkey breast in each half of pita with half of the olive mixture and quarter cup of greens. Keep in check the sodium quantity of the other ingredients while using olives in your recipes.

Did you know?

The important nutrients found in green and black olives include Vitamin E, Lignans, Coumaric acids and tyrosols.

121. Peppered Bacon Chickoli

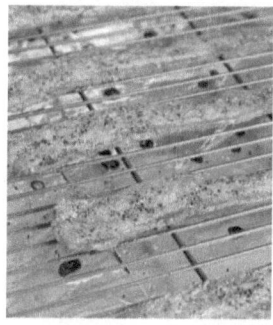

This meal is particularly good for weight loss because of the inclusion of pepper, which, as are most spices, is good for weight loss endeavors because it helps to speed up metabolism.

Ingredients (2 servings)

- 1/2 pound of broccoli

- 1/2 pound of peppered bacon strips
- 2 large chicken breasts

Method

1. Butter the slow cooker and put the bacon strips in layers. Add a layer of broccoli then a chicken breast. Put a second layer of bacon, followed by broccoli and then the last breast. Put last bacon layer and last broccoli layer and add 1½ cups of water. Cook on low for five to six hours.

Did you know?

Broccoli has all three of beneficial components found in vegetables, one of which, indole-3-carbinol is known to prevent hormone related cancers like prostate and breast cancers.

122. Slow Cooked Low Carb Mexi Chicken

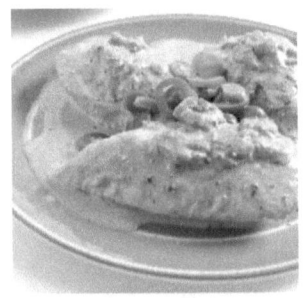

Eating chicken is good for a weight loss diet because unlike other meat types like beef and pork, it is low in fat but high in protein. That makes this meal highly beneficial.

Ingredients (one serving)

- 8 ounces chicken breasts
- 2 teaspoons taco seasoning
- ½ cup salsa
- 1 cup grated medium/ low fat cheddar cheese

Method

1. Spray the base and the sides of the slow cooker with non-stick spray. Season the chicken generously with taco seasoning on both sides and

spoon salsa on top. Place in the slow cooker and cook on low for 5¾ hours. Open pot and sprinkle cheese evenly on the breasts. Close pot and cook for a further 15 minutes

Did you know?

Chicken is niacin rich and the niacin is essential for brain health and may have protective factors against Alzheimer's disease and dementia.

123. Slow Cooker Carnitas

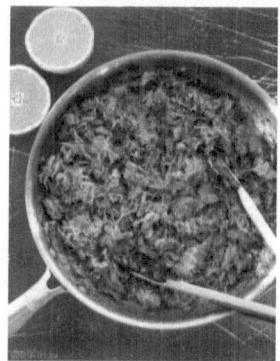

Pork is the main ingredient in this Mexican meal. This makes the meal good for weight loss because pork has high protein content and no carbohydrates. On the other hand, garlic is beneficial as it has anti-bacterial, anti-fungal and anti-oxidant properties.

Ingredients (4 servings)

- 2 pounds boneless pork cut into 5 or 6 pieces
- 1¼ teaspoon salt
- 1 teaspoon chili powder and one teaspoon cumin
- 1 bay leaf
- 4 thinly sliced garlic cloves
- 1 chopped medium sized onion

Method

1. Rub the pre-mixed dry ingredients into the meat. Place the meat as a single layer in a buttered cock pot. Place the bay leaf then sprinkle the onions and garlic on top. Cook on low heat for 5 to 6 hours. Place meat in an oven dish to brown (optional).

Did you know?

Cumin is the second most popular spice in the world, after black pepper. It contains 'thymol', an acid production stomach stimulating compound which enables the body to get maximum benefits from food.

124. Beef and Vegetable Parmesan

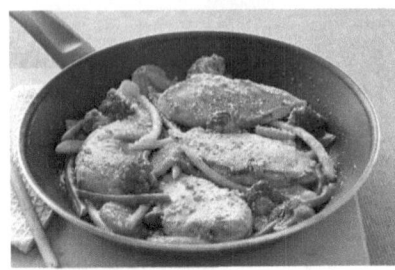

This tasty dish has easily available ingredients and helps lose weight because it has a total of between 2225 and 2300kj per serving. It has net carbs of 7g per serving and these figures will push you forward to your desired weight loss goal.

Ingredients (Serves 2)

- 1-pound boneless beef sirloin
- 4 cups broccoli florets
- 2 cups cauliflower florets
- 5 tablespoons shredded parmesan cheese
- 2-3 tablespoons olive oil
- Salt and freshly ground pepper

Method

1. Cut beef into sizable pieces. Sprinkle seasoning. Put a layer of the vegetables on the crock pot. Place the meat on top and add the remaining vegetables on the sides and on top of the meat. Add about 50 milliliters of water. Cook on medium heat for 3-4 hours. Sprinkle the cheese on top before serving.

Did you know?

Olive oil is rich in the anti-oxidant hydroxytyrosol. Anti-oxidants help protect the body against the damage caused by free radicals.

125. Slow Cooked Tilapia Parmesan

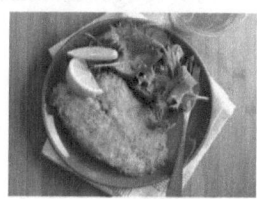

Tilapia is the main ingredient in this dish and it helps you lose weight because it has no carbohydrates, no sugar and very little fat and therefore very little calorie count.

Ingredients (serves 4)

- 2 pounds tilapia
- 2 ounces parmesan cheese
- ¼ cup butter
- 3 tablespoons mayonnaise
- ¼ teaspoon each of garlic powder and pepper
- A small onion, chopped
- Choice seasoning

Method

1. Spray non-stick spray at the base of the crock pot. Carefully place the fish and season lightly. Mix all the other ingredients except cheese and spoon mixture on top of fish. Cook on low heat for three hours. Add the cheese on top and cook for a further hour.

Did you know?

Tilapia is a good source of Omega 3 fatty acids which can help you maintain a healthy blood pressure while keeping many diseases at bay.

126. Slow Cooker Thai Curry Beef

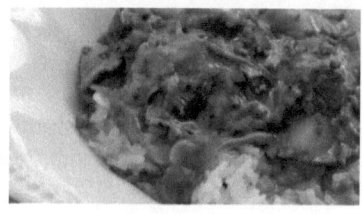

This dish has the benefits of protein from the beef and the mushrooms. The high protein value keeps you full for longer and keeps hunger pangs at bay.

Ingredients (serves 4)

- 4 teaspoons red/ green Thai curry paste
- 14 ounces can coconut milk
- 3 tablespoons fish or soy sauce
- 2 pounds steak or chuck roast in sizable pieces
- 8 ounces mushrooms
- Medium onion and carrot both sliced thinly
- 10 ounces cauliflower florets
- 2 teaspoons salt
- ½ teaspoon pepper
- 12 ounces trimmed fresh green beans

Method

1. Whisk the paste, milk and sauce in the slow cooker. Add the remaining ingredients except beans and stir to ensure sauce coats everything. Add the beans but do not mix. Cook on low heat for 8 hours, in the last 30 minutes, stir in the beans at ten-minute intervals.

Did you know?

Cauliflower is packed with health benefits including better digestion and it also contains allicin, which has been found to reduce the occurrence of stroke and heart disease.

127. Slow Cooked Stuffed Gammon

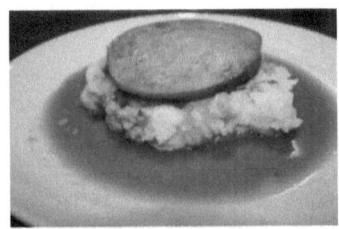

The main ingredient in this dish is beef, and beef is one of the greatest sources of protein. Beef will help you get to the desired amount of proteins per day and because it has no carbs, you can be sure you keep on track of your desired weight loss endeavor.

Ingredients (serves 5-8)

- 4 pounds boneless gammon
- 1 1 tablespoon oil
- 2 tablespoons curry paste
- 1 cup cooked couscous
- 1 cup dried apples, chopped
- 1 cup dried cranberries
- ½ cup each of pine nuts and maple syrup
- 2 tablespoons vegetable stock
- 2 tablespoon course mustard
- Salt and pepper

Method

1. Grease the crock pot. Make a big hole in the center of the gammon using a flat, sharp knife. Heat oil in a saucepan and add curry, couscous, apples, cranberries and nuts. Season well, remove from the pan and leave to cool. Stuff into gammon and secure with kitchen string. Place in crock pot. Close and cook for 6 hours on low heat. In a bowl, combine syrup, stock and mustard. Pour over gammon and cook again for two hours. Place in oven to brown.

Did you know?

Berries are good for your memory. They contain flavonoids which can improve memory, learning and general cognitive function including reasoning, decision making and verbal comprehension.

128. Slow Cooker Breakfast Casserole

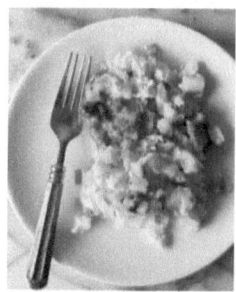

This dish is a filling breakfast dish that has essential nutrients to keep you going and fulfilled for several hours.

Ingredients (5 servings)

- ½ pound ground sausage, browned and drained
- 6 large eggs
- ½ cup milk
- 1-pound frozen hash-browns
- ½ cup salsa
- ½ cup grated cheddar cheese
- ½ pound potatoes
- Salt and pepper to taste

Method

1. Spray non-stick cooking spray into the crock pot. Thoroughly mix together beaten eggs, milk and the salt and pepper before pouring into the cooker. Add the remaining ingredients and stir a little. Cook on low heat for six hours until mixture sets at the center.

Did you know?

Eggs are good for alertness. The protein in egg is an essential component of neurotransmitters like dopamine and norepinephrine which help communication between brain cells.

129. Apple Cinnamon Slow Cooker Oatmeal

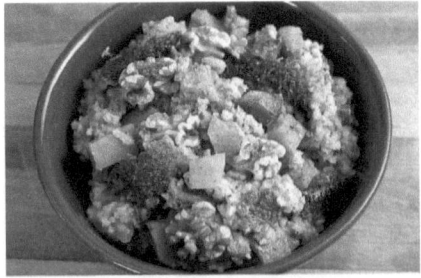

This dish has great benefits for low carb induced weight loss because it has very little net cards, little if any fat and only natural sugars from the apples.

Ingredients (4 servings)

- 2 peeled and sliced apples
- 1 teaspoon cinnamon
- ⅓ cup brown sugar

- 2 cups oats, steel-cut
- 4 cups water
- A little salt to taste

Method

1. Line the base of your slow cooker. Slice the apples at the bottom of the cooker. Pour cinnamon and brown sugar on the apples and stir to mix. Pour oats, salt and the water and do not mix again. Cook overnight, 8-9 hours on low. Stir before you serve.

Did you know?

Oats are great for concentration. They are a good source of fiber and are a low GI grain. They provide glucose which can fuel your body for a long time which is not the case with fast released sugary foods.

130. Slow Cooker Sausage and Egg Breakfast Casserole

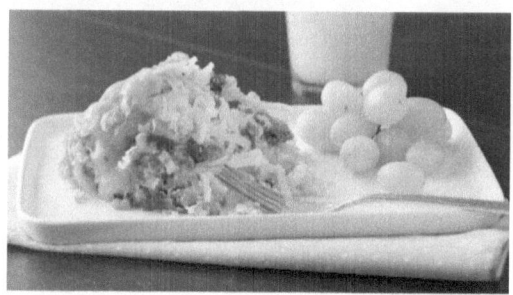

This dish's main advantages lie in its filling nature. Sausage and broccoli makes you so full that you will not get hunger pangs before your next planned meal. Each serving has 4.21 g net carbs so you have no fear of going overboard.

Ingredients (6 servings)

- 1 medium head broccoli, chopped
- 12 ounces pork sausages, cooked and sliced
- 1 cup shredded cheddar cheese
- 10 eggs
- ¾ cup whipping cream
- 2 garlic cloves, minced
- ½ teaspoon salt and ¼ teaspoon pepper

Method

1. Grease the interior of your slow cooker well. Layer half of broccoli, half the sausage and half the cheese into the pot and repeat with the remaining halves. Whisk together the remaining ingredients and well mixed. Gently pour into the crock pot on top of the other ingredients. Cover and cook on high for 2-3 hours. It has to brown on the edges and the center has to set.

Did you know?

Broccoli is termed a miracle food because of the many health benefits it has. Broccoli contains beta carotene and vitamin C, important anti-oxidants linked to reduced risk of many conditions like cataracts and heart disease among several.

131. Savory Bean Cake

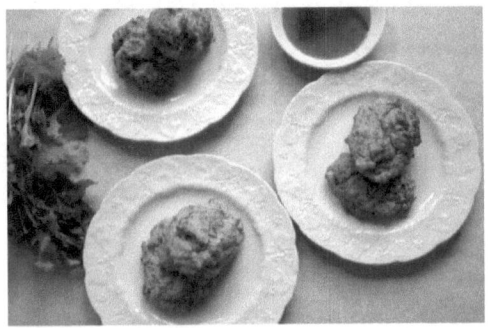

The egg and beans combination in this dish is very good for weight loss. These two ingredients provide proteins which make you full for some time at the same time giving you other health benefits.

Ingredients (4 servings)

- 3 cups black-eyed beans
- 1 onion, peeled
- 1 teaspoon curry paste
- 1 stock cube
- 3 tablespoons fresh coriander
- 4 tablespoons butter, melted
- 1 cup self-raising floor
- 4 eggs, boiled

Method

1. Soak beans for 8-10 hours. Rinse well and put into blender and blend until smooth, remove from blender. Put onions, pepper, curry paste, stock cube, coriander and butter into blender and blend until smooth. Mix well with beans and add flour, mix.

2. Place non-stick cooking paper in crock pot and put half the blended mixture on the base (preferably the smallest crock pot). Add the eggs and cover with remaining mixture. Close pot and cook on low for three hours.

Did you know?

Beans provide a slow release of glucose which enables a steady supply of energy to make the brain function at its best. Beans contain folate which is essential for brain health because it helps by reducing the levels homocysteine, an amino acid which can reduce brain function.

132. Slow Cooked Fish Cakes

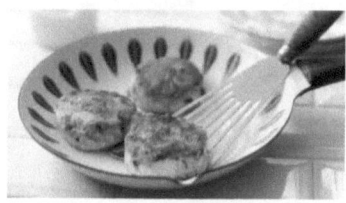

White fish is a proven weight loss assisting ingredient. Hake is a source of Omega 3 fatty acids so this gives this dish all the benefits of Omega 3 fatty acids including but not limited to controlling heart disease, cholesterol and the protection against the accumulation of the Alzheimer's disease linked protein.

Ingredients (6 servings)

- 1-pound hake or whiting steaks
- 2 potatoes, cooked and mashed
- I onion, grated
- 3 tablespoons chopped parsley
- 2 teaspoons lemon juice
- 2 beaten eggs
- 4 tablespoons flour
- Salt and pepper

Method

1. Grease your crock pot, preferably one with a large base. Put fish into blender and blend slightly. Mix fish with mashed potato, onions, parsley, lemon juice, eggs, flour, salt and pepper. Shape the mixture into six cakes.

2. Sprinkle flour on a board and roll the fish cakes. Place individually in crock pot. Close and cook on low for six hours. Put on oven rake and grill for a minute or two to brown.

Did you know?

Though high in carbohydrates, potatoes in moderation are good for keeping inflammation down. Nutrients like vitamin C, B and potassium are good for relieving inflammation of the intestines and the digestive system. Potatoes are soft; are easy to digest therefore making them good for those with mouth ulcers.

133. Low Carb Slow Cooker Jambalaya

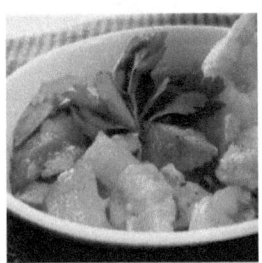

This dish is rich in spices and spices are known for greatly aiding weight loss. Spices are known to speed up metabolism which in turn helps you lose weight faster.

Ingredients (2-3 servings)

- 1 cup chopped onion
- 1 cup chopped green pepper
- 1 cup chopped celery
- 2 garlic cloves, minced
- 1 28 ounces can un-drained diced tomatoes
- ¾ pound cooked prawns
- 2 cups turkey sausage or smoked sausage
- ¼ teaspoon each of hot sauce and pepper

- ½ teaspoon each of salt and dried thyme
- 1 tablespoon dried parsley

Method

1. Add all ingredients except prawns and stir well. Cook on high for 3-4 hours. Add prawns to crock pot for the last 15 minutes of cooking time.

Did you know?

That tomato is not a vegetable but a fruit and that it helps keep you focused. Red and purple fruits and foods contain the phytochemical anthocyanin which helps you keep your memory sharp and fully focused. It also has the potential of positive mood creation and overall clarity.

134. Low Carb Crock Pot Chili

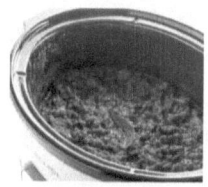

This dish is amazing and great for the desired weight loss goal. The mixture of different spices, each with its own health benefit is such that the dish becomes a conglomeration of health and weight loss benefits.

Ingredients (serves 4)

- 1-pound lean ground beef, browned and drained
- 1 cup chopped inion
- 3 stalks celery, diced
- 2 cloves garlic, minced
- 1 14 ounces can diced tomato with juice
- 1 8 ounces can tomato sauce
- 1 14 ounces can low sodium beef broth
- 1 cup hot water
- 1½ teaspoon chili powder
- ½ teaspoon each of cumin, oregano and paprika
- Dash of cayenne pepper
- 1 teaspoon each of salt and black pepper

Method

1. Mix all the ingredients in the crock pot. Cook on low heat for 6-8 hours.

Did you know?

Oregano is one of the oldest known culinary and medicinal herbs. It has literally been used in cooking and medicine for thousands of years and it contains several known health benefits. It has anti-oxidant and anti-bacterial properties.

135. Cheesy Cauliflower Soup

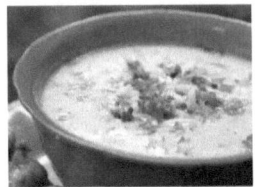

This is one of the most weight loss friendly soups you can ever have. It has only 6 calories per serving which will ensure that you certainly head in the right weight loss direction.

Ingredients (serves 4)

- 1 cauliflower head, chopped
- 1 onion, chopped
- 1 stalk celery, chopped
- 4 cups chicken stock
- ½ teaspoon Worcestershire sauce
- 1 cup heavy cream
- 2 cups American cheese, shredded
- Chopped chives
- Salt and pepper to taste.

Method

1. Put cauliflower, onion, celery and stock in a crock pot. Cover and cook on low for 6-8 hours. Puree the mixture and return to pot. Add cream, Worcestershire sauce, cheese, salt and pepper to the mixture and stir to mix. Turn heat to high and cook until hot and melted.

Did you know?

Cauliflower helps in cancer prevention. Cauliflower is a cruciferous vegetable and this family of vegetables is linked to significant reduction in risk of cancer, especially ovarian cancer, prostate cancer, breast cancer, colon cancer and bladder cancer.

136. Winter Vegetable Soup

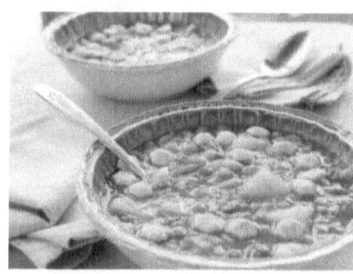

The main ingredient in this dish is beef, and beef is one of the greatest sources of protein. Beef will help you get to the desired amount of proteins per day and because it has no carbs, you can be sure you keep on track of your desired weight loss endeavor.

Ingredients (serves 4)

- 2 pounds ground chuck, browned and drained
- 1 large tomato can
- 1 large can tomato sauce
- 1 package dry onion soup mix
- 1 can each of beef broth and water
- 1 package frozen mixed vegetables

Method

1. Mix all the ingredients in crock pot. Close pot and cook on low for 8-9 hours.

Did you know?

Tomato helps keep you focused. Red and purple foods contain the phytochemical anthocyanin which helps you keep your memory sharp and fully focused. It also has the potential of positive mood creation and overall clarity of mind. You can cook it or enjoy it raw and still get the same benefits.

137. Serene Day Beef Soup

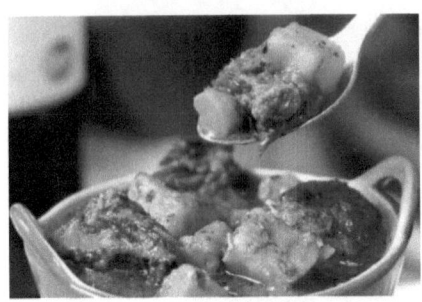

The main ingredient in this dish is beef, and with beef you cannot go wrong because it is one of the greatest sources of protein. Beef helps you get to the desired amount of proteins per day because that is the main nutrient is it; and because it has no carbs, you can be sure you keep on track of your desired weight loss endeavor.

Ingredients (5-7 servings)

- 2 pounds beef cut into bite sized pieces
- 2 cans 14 ounces beef broth
- 1 undrained 14 ounces can diced tomatoes with garlic and onions
- 1 cup water
- 1 teaspoon salt
- 1 teaspoon crushed Italian seasoning
- ½ teaspoon pepper
- 4 cups frozen vegetables
- 1 cup uncooked low carb pasta

Method

1. Combine beef, broth, tomatoes, water, salt, Italian seasoning and pepper to crock and mix well. Cover and cook on high for 5 hours. Stir in vegetables and pasta. Cook covered for 1 hour to 1½ hours and stir before serving.

Did you know?

Garlic has been used in food and medicine for more than five thousand years, is one of the most common ingredients in Indian food and has up to 15 health benefits including lowering blood pressure and detoxification. It is also a source of selenium.

138. Creamy Chicken and Peppers Enchilada

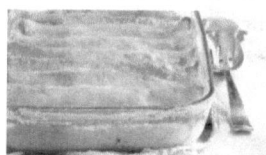

One of the main ingredients in this dish is chicken and chicken is a good source of lean protein. It is good to eat for weight loss because it is lower in fat and calories compared to other types of meat.

Ingredients (serves 4)

- 2 pounds chicken breasts
- ½ can enchilada sauce
- 2 ounces chopped green chilies
- 1 each of small green and red pepper, chopped
- 8-ounce package cream cheese, cut into cubes and softened
- 2 cups shredded cheddar cheese

Method

1. Place chicken, enchilada sauce and chilies in a large slow cooker. Cover and cook on low heat about 8-10 hours. Stir in peppers, cream cheese and cheddar cheese. Cover crock pot and cook on low heat for 30-45 minutes until cheese is melted. Stir once or twice.

Did you know?

Chili peppers might be very hot, but they are still one of the most common spices throughout the world. The chili plant originates from the Central American region where it was used as one of the main spice ingredients in Mexican dishes for several hundred years. It was introduced to the rest of the world by Portuguese and Spanish explorers in the 16th and 17th centuries.

139. Slow Cooked Tamale Bake

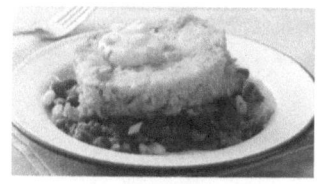

Beef is the main ingredient in this dish. It helps you get to the desired amount of proteins per day because that is the main nutrient is it; and because it has no carbohydrates, you can be sure you keep in sight of your desired weight loss effort.

Ingredients (5-6 servings)

- 1½ pounds ground beef
- 1 onion, chopped
- 2 garlic cloves, minced
- 10-ounce enchilada sauce
- 1 package Atkins corn muffin mix
- 1/3 cup heavy cream
- 2 tablespoons melted butter
- 1 egg
- ¾ cup shredded Colby Cheese
- 4 ounces can, undrained
- chopped green chilies
- ½ cup each of salsa and sour cream

Method

1. Use non-stick skillet to cook ground beef, onion and garlic over medium heat until meat is cooked. Drain thoroughly and stir in enchilada sauce. Pour into crock pot. Separately mix together corn muffin mix, cream, butter and egg just until combined. Add cheese and can chilies. Spoon over beef in crock pot. Cover pot and cook on low for 6-7 hours.

What Makes Garlic So Popular?

Garlic has been used in food and medicine for more than five thousand years, is one of the most common ingredients in Indian food and has up to 15 health benefits including lowering blood pressure and detoxification. It is also a source of selenium which has anti-oxidant properties.

140. Cabbage Roll Stew

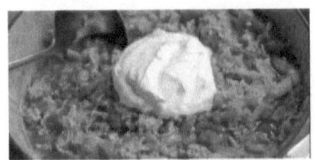

This dish has the potential to aid in weight loss. The protein it provides from the beef keeps you full for a long time and prevents hunger pangs. In addition, the protein in beef enables you to meet you daily protein requirement without a struggle.

Ingredients (4 servings)

- 1-pound lean ground beef
- 1 medium onion, chopped
- 14 ounces stewed tomatoes
- 14 ounces tomato sauce
- 1 tablespoon each of minced garlic
- Worcestershire sauce
- 1 cup chicken broth
- 1 teaspoon pepper
- ½ teaspoon hot pepper
- ½ cabbage head, chopped

Method

1. Brown beef and onions in a pot. Place all ingredients except cabbage in crock pot and mix well. Add beef mixture then cabbage and cook on low for 5-6 hours.

Did you know?

Cabbage is a cruciferous vegetable and this family of vegetables is linked to significant reduction in risk of cancer, especially ovarian cancer, prostate cancer, breast cancer, colon cancer and bladder cancer. In addition, cabbage can stop running tummies and can improve appetite.

141. Slow Cooker Boston Baked Beans

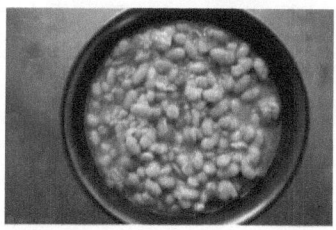

Write a little summary about why this dish is healthy and helps with the proposed solution. Maybe address one or two of the key ingredients.

Ingredients (16 servings)

- 4 cups uncooked white beans
- 2 cups onion chopped
- 4 slices bacon, chopped
- ¼ cup low sugar ketchup
- 1/3 cup molasses
- 12 packet Krisda stevia
- 1 teaspoon pepper
- 1 tablespoon Worcestershire
- 2 tablespoon mustard
- 6 cups water

Method

1. Soak beans overnight. Drain and rinse beans and put in crock pot with all the other ingredients. Cook on high for 8-9 hours.

Did you know?

¼ to ½ a cup of cooked legumes (beans is a type of legumes) provides about 100 micrograms of folate which is essential for brain health as it helps to reduce levels of homocysteine, an amino acid which can impair brain functions. There are reports of low folate levels being linked to depression.

142. Spinach, artichoke and Kale Dip

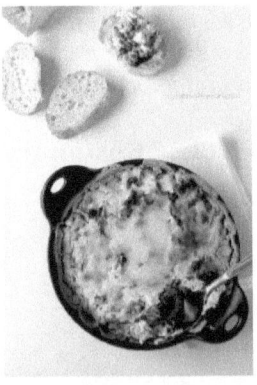

Every ingredient in this dish is nutrient packed and that makes the dish highly nutritious. The dish is low in calories and net carbs and contains many health benefits from the nutritious ingredients.

Ingredients (20 servings)

- 2-3 garlic cloves
- ½ onion
- 2 14 ounces cans artichoke hearts
- 10 ounces each of chopped kale and spinach
- 1 cup each of parmesan cheese, shredded mozzarella, no fat Greek yogurt
- ¾ cup low fat sour cream
- ¼ cup low fat mayo
- Salt and pepper

Method

1. Use food processor to chop garlic, artichokes and onion into smaller pieces. Add everything to crock pot and stir. Cook on high for 4 hours. Season with salt and pepper as desired.

Did you know?

Spinach is one of the best sources of potassium in the diet. It also contains calcium, iron, magnesium and even protein. Spinach as a source of iron determines how efficiently your body uses energy.

143. Sweet Potato Breakfast Casserole

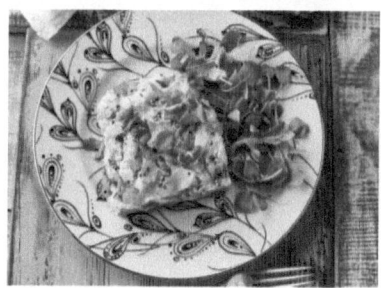

Whether you like sweet potatoes or not, you will love staring your day with this satisfying meal.

Ingredients

- 1-pound ground meat of your choice
- ½ tsp garlic powder
- 1 tsp salt

- ¼ tsp thyme
- ¼ tsp sage
- 1/8 tsp red pepper
- 4 cups peeled sweet potatoes, cubed
- 1 bell pepper, diced
- 1 small onion, diced
- 8 eggs
- ½ cup milk
- Salt and pepper

Method

1. Preheat oven to 350 degrees. Brown ground meat with seasonings and onion. Place cubed sweet potatoes in a 9x13 pan. Broil for 10 minutes. Place browned meat over sweet potatoes. Whisk together eggs and milk with salt and pepper. Pour the egg mixture over meat and potatoes. Bake for 20-30 minutes.

Notes

You can make this recipe the night before and refrigerate. Put the prepared pan in a cold oven set at 350 degrees and bake for 40 minutes. The leftovers are great, too!

144. Wheat-Free Frittata

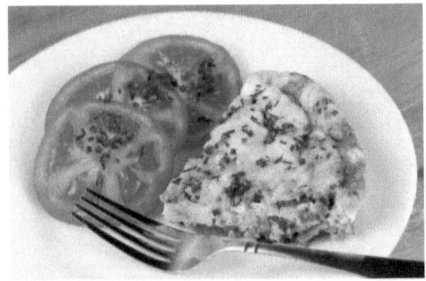

This recipe is simple and quick. You can use the basic recipe and throw in whatever ingredients you have on hand.

Ingredients

- 2 cups broccoli, chopped
- ¼ - ½ Bacon, ham, or sausage, chopped
- 2 tomatoes, chopped

- 5 eggs, beaten
- ¼ cup milk
- 1 tsp garlic
- Salt and pepper
- ¼ cup cheese of your choice, shredded

Method

1. Microwave broccoli with 2 T water for 3 minutes. Grease a pie plate and layer the broccoli and other veggies. Mix eggs, milk, and spices. Pour over veggies in pie plate. Sprinkle with grated cheese. Bake at 350 degrees for 30-35 minutes.

Notes

This dish makes great left-overs.

145. Pancakes

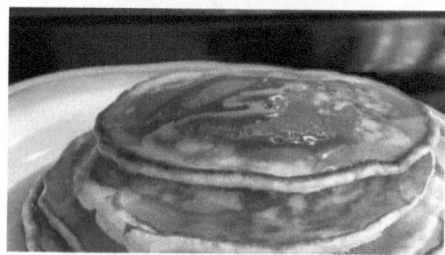

Everybody loves pancakes on a Saturday morning. Thanks to this recipe, you no longer have to feel sluggish the rest of the day after eating them. No need to use store bought coconut flour, just grind coconut flakes in a blender or food processor.

Ingredients

- 2 eggs, beaten
- 1 cup milk
- 1 tsp vanilla
- 1 cup almond flour
- ¼ cup coconut flour
- ¼ cup sugar
- 2 tsp baking powder
- ½ tsp salt

Method

1. Combine dry ingredients. Combine wet ingredients. Pour wet ingredients into dry ingredients and mix. Pour by ¼ cup portions onto hot griddle. Flip when bubbles appear.

Notes

You can add a smashed banana, blueberries, or chocolate chips.

146. Oatmeal Banana Bake

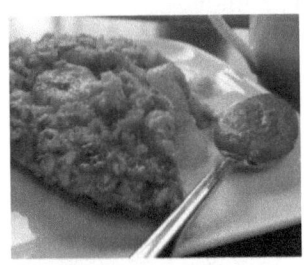

Good for breakfast or a snack any time of day.

Ingredients

- 1 ¼ cup rolled oats
- ¾ cup milk
- ½ cup brown sugar
- 1/3 cup oil
- 2 large bananas, mashed
- 1 egg, beaten
- 1 ½ cup oat flour
- ½ tsp cinnamon
- ½ tsp nutmeg
- ½ tsp salt
- 1 tsp baking soda
- 2 tsp baking powder

Method

1. Grease an 8-inch baking pan. Mix dry ingredients. Mix eggs, banana, milk, and oil. Pour mixture into dry ingredients, mix well. Spread evenly in pan. Bake at 350 degrees for 30-40 minutes.

Notes

½ cup chopped walnuts are a great addition to this recipe.

147. Biscuits

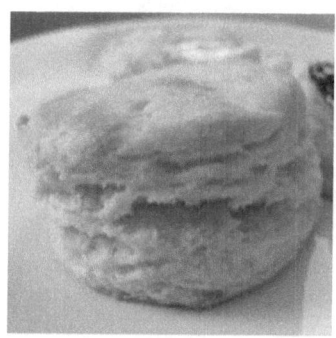

These fluffy biscuits can be served warm with butter or jelly, or topped with sausage gravy. (Recipe follows.)

Ingredients

- 1 cup almond flour
- 1 tsp baking powder
- ½ tsp salt
- 2 tbsp. cold butter
- 3 eggs, whites only

Method

1. Mix flour salt and baking soda. Add butter and mix with your fingers or a pastry cutter until crumbly. Whisk the egg whites for about 30 seconds, until frothy. Combine eggs with flour mixture. Refrigerate for 20 minutes. Use a spoon to drop 4-6 biscuits on a greased pan. Bake at 400 degrees until lightly browned.

Notes

If you want more muffins, mix another batch rather than trying to double the recipe. Uncooked biscuit round can be frozen for later use.

Freeze on a baking sheet until solid and then put them in a bag in the freezer. Thaw in the fridge for two hours when you are ready to use them.

148. Biscuit Gravy

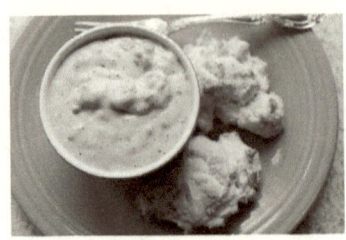

Pour this gravy over your homemade biscuits and feel like you're in the south no matter where you live.

Ingredients

- ½ pound ground sausage
- ¼ tsp black pepper
- ¼ tsp salt
- 2 tbsp. almond flour
- 1 tbsp. butter
- 2 cups whole milk

Method

1. Brown sausage in a pan. Mix flour well with milk. Add spices, milk, and butter to browned meat. Mix well. Simmer covered for 10 minutes on low heat. Pour over prepared biscuits.

149. Cauliflower Pizza Crust

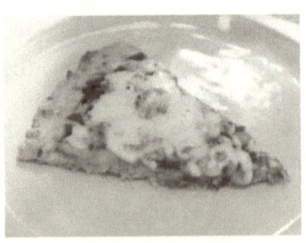

You may be skeptical, but push past your skepticism and the reward is great.

Ingredients

- 1 small head cauliflower
- ¼ cup parmesan cheese

- ¼ cup mozzarella cheese
- ¼ tsp salt
- 1 tsp Italian spice
- ½ tsp garlic powder
- 1 egg

Method

1. Wash cauliflower and cut off florets. Pulse florets in food processor until flaky. Cook in microwave for four minutes. Add cheeses, spices, and almond meal. Mix. Add egg and mix. Form the dough into a crust and set on a greased baking sheet. Bake at 400 degrees for 8-11 minutes or until browned. Add whatever toppings you like and bake for another 8-10 minutes.

Notes

Pizza night no longer means eating lots of grain filled crust. And with this crust, you won't miss it a bit.

150. Flat Bread

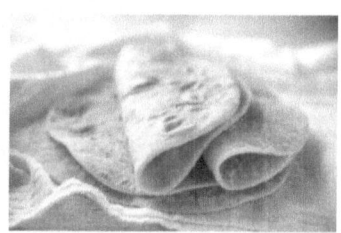

Flat bread is great for sandwiches or with your favorite soup or pasta dish. And this wheat free version is just as good as the grain laden kind.

Ingredients

- 4 cups almond flour
- 2 cups warm water
- 2 ½ tsp yeast
- 1 tsp salt

Method

1. In a large bowl, combine warm water, yeast, and salt. Cover and let rest for 2 hours. Divide dough into 12 sections. Flatten into 6-inch

rounds. Place one round on a hot griddle. Cook until it bubbles. Turn and cook for 1-2 more minutes. Repeat with remaining rounds.

Notes

The rounds can be stored in a plastic bag in the refrigerator for up to two weeks before cooking.

151. Enchilada Casserole

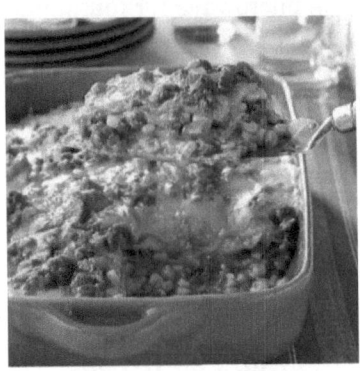

This is a simple dish to which you can add as many veggies as you like.

Ingredients

- 1 package wheat free corn tortillas
- 1-pound ground meat of your choice
- ½ tbsp. oil
- ½ cup onion, chopped
- 1 can Enchilada sauce
- 2 cups cheese, grated

Method

1. Brown ground meat and onions in a pan. Layer corn tortillas, meat, enchilada sauce and cheese. Top with cheese. Bake at 350 degrees for 45-60 minutes or until cheese bubbles around the edges.

Notes

If you like spicy food, add chopped peppers or red pepper flakes to the meat mixture.

152. Chicken and Dumplings

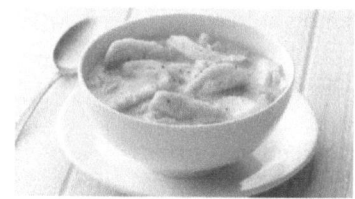

If you keep frozen biscuit rounds and chopped cooked chicken in the freezer, you can pull them out in the morning and have them ready for this recipe when you get home in the evening. That makes it super simple.

Ingredients

- Biscuit dough, uncooked.
- 6 cups chicken stock
- 2 cooked chicken breasts, cubed
- 1/3 cup shredded carrots
- 1/3 cup minced celery
- 1 cup heavy cream
- Salt and pepper
- 3 T parsley, chopped

Method

1. Place the chicken stock, chicken, carrots, and celery in a stock pot and bring to a boil. Add uncooked biscuit dough to boiling liquid and reduce to a simmer. Stir in cream, salt and pepper. Cover and cook 6-8 minutes. Ladle into bowl and sprinkle with parsley.

Note

See the biscuit recipe in this book for the biscuit dough.

153. Chicken Strips

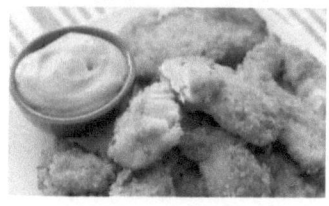

Giving up wheat doesn't mean you have to give up old favorites, like chicken strips. This recipe makes the old favorite healthy and delicious. Coconut oil is best for cooking at high temperatures.

Ingredients

- 4 chicken breasts, sliced into strips
- 2 eggs
- 1 tbsp. water
- ¾ cup almond flour
- ½ tsp salt
- ¼ tsp pepper
- 1 cup coconut oil

Method

1. Whisk the eggs and water together in a bowl. In another bowl, combine dry ingredients. Heat coconut oil over medium heat in a skillet. Dip chicken in egg mixture, and then in the flour mixture, coating completely. Cook in hot coconut oil, turning as needed to brown all sides. Place cooked chicken strips on paper towel.

Notes

Serve these up with your favorite dipping sauce. Buffalo or Ranch dressing works nicely.

154. Quinoa Casserole

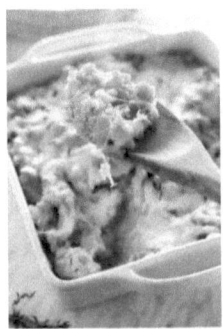

Quinoa is an ancient grain which is low on the glycemic index, provides eight essential amino acids, and is one of the best sources of protein in the vegetable kingdom.

Ingredients

- 1 bag of broccoli florets, chopped
- 1 ½ cups quinoa, cooked according to package instructions and cooled
- 3 eggs
- 1 cup low-fat cottage cheese
- 3 tbsp. almond flour
- Salt and pepper
- ½ cup parmesan cheese, shredded

Method

1. Heat broccoli in a saucepan. Beat eggs and add in quinoa, cottage cheese, almond flour, and salt and pepper. Add cooked broccoli. Place mixture in a greased casserole dish. Bake at 350 degrees for 35 minutes. Top with parmesan cheese and serve.

Notes

Use this casserole as a main dish and serve the left-overs as a side dish.

155. Flaxseed Wraps

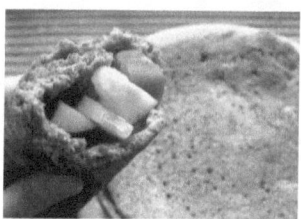

Flaxseed is high in omega 3 fatty acids and high in fiber. It can be purchased already ground into meal or as seeds which you can grind at home.

Ingredients

- ¼ cup flax meal
- ¾ tsp baking powder
- ¼ tsp garlic
- ¼ tsp salt
- 1 tbsp. water
- 1 egg, beaten
- 1 tbsp. coconut oil, melted

Method

1. Combine all ingredients. Heat a skillet over medium-high heat. Pour batter evenly into pan. Cook for 3-4 minutes and remove from pan. Fill these healthy wraps with your favorite sandwich fixings or scrambled eggs and cheese.

156. Macaroni and Cheese

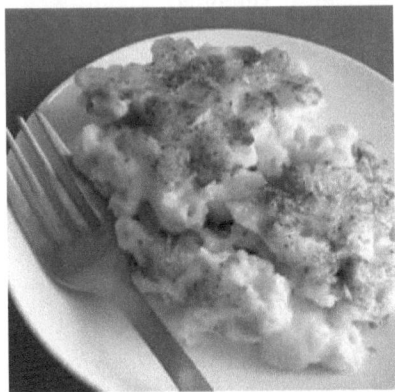

One pot. No wheat. 15 minutes to make. Enough said.

Ingredients

- 3 cups wheat free pasta
- 2 ¼ cup milk
- 2 cups water
- 1 tsp salt
- 2 cups cheddar cheese, grated
- Salt and pepper

Method

1. Put all ingredients, except the cheese, into a large saucepan. Bring to a boil over medium heat. Simmer 8 minutes, or until pasta is cooked al-dente. Stir in the cheese.

Notes

Alternatives to wheat pasta are readily available in stores, making it possible to make all your pasta dishes wheat free.

157. Meatloaf

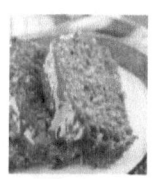

Many meatloaf recipes call for unhealthy ingredients like brown sugar or saltine crackers. This is a much healthier version. And you won't miss the crackers at all.

Ingredients

- 2 pounds ground beef
- 2 eggs
- 1 medium onion, diced
- 1 tsp onion powder
- 1 tsp garlic powder
- 1 tsp salt
- ¼ tsp nutmeg
- ½ tsp ground mustard
- 3 cloves garlic, minced
- 1 tbsp. butter

Method

1. Sauté onions and garlic in butter. Combine all ingredients. Form into a loaf and place in a greased, glass loaf pan. Bake at 350 degrees for 50 minutes. Let sit for 5 minutes before serving.

Notes

Meatloaf goes great with the cauliflower mashed potatoes in the next recipe.

158. Cauliflower Mashed Potatoes

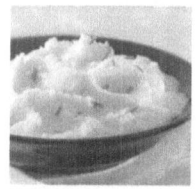

The texture is right. The taste is right. And no one will know it's not made with unhealthy white potatoes.

Ingredients

- 1 head cauliflower, florets only
- ¼ cup butter
- ½ cup sour cream
- 1 tsp garlic powder
- Salt and pepper

Method

1. Steam cauliflower until very soft. Let cool for 15-20 minutes. Place all ingredients in a food processor and pulse until smooth. Heat and serve.

159. Crusty Chicken Casserole

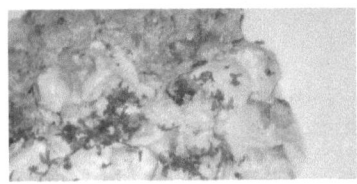

This simple one pan dish is sure to satisfy.

Ingredients

- 3 chicken breasts, cubed
- 1 cup chicken broth
- 1 tsp garlic powder
- 1 tsp onion powder
- ¼ tsp chili pepper
- ¼ tsp salt
- 6 ounces cream cheese, cubed
- 1 cup cheddar cheese, shredded

For the Crust

- ½ cup almond flour
- ¼ cup flax meal
- ¼ cup milk

- 2 eggs
- 1 tsp baking powder

Method

1. Dice chicken and place in the bottom of a casserole dish. Pour in chicken broth. Sprinkle seasonings and cream cheese on top. Sprinkle shredded cheese. Mix crust ingredients. Spread crust evenly over chicken. Bake at 350 degrees for 40 minutes.

Notes

This will be, hands down, the best crusty, cheesy chicken dish you have ever made.

160. Cheese Crackers

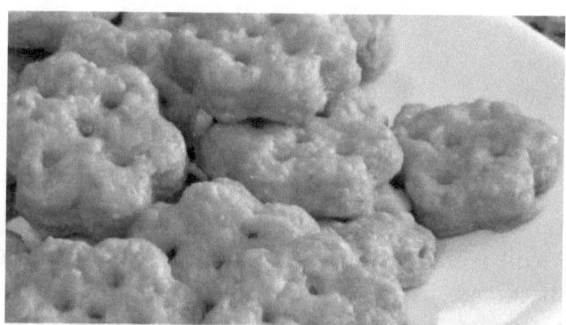

Crispy, delicious, and easy.

Ingredients

- Cheese of your choice, grated
- Seasonings of your choice such as garlic or red pepper flakes

Method

1. Place small piles of cheese on parchment paper. Microwave for 1 minute.

Notes

Dip these crispy chips in sour cream for a wonderful wheat free snack.

161. Pretzels

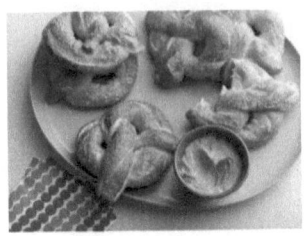

Again, almond flour saves us from the wheat.

Ingredients

- 2 eggs, beaten
- 1 ½ cups almond flour
- ½ tsp salt
- 1 tbsp. butter
- 1 tsp water
- Coarse salt

Method

1. Mix almond flour, salt, and butter. Pour in 1 beaten eggs and mix into dough. Roll a chunk of dough into a thin strip about 6 inched long. Place the dough in pretzel form on a greased baking sheet. Bake at 350 degrees for ten minutes. Turn pretzels over, brush with the other egg and sprinkle with coarse salt. Bake at 400 degrees for 5 minutes. Let cool.

Notes

These pretzels are soft and delicious and great with a bit of mustard for dipping.

162. Thai Salmon Soup

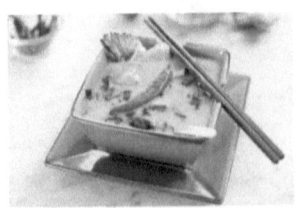

Keep canned salmon on hand so you can make this dish anytime.

Ingredients

- 1 can coconut milk
- 1 can salmon
- 1 tbsp. salt
- 2 tsp virgin coconut oil
- Water, as needed
- 1 tsp basil
- ½ tsp ginger

Method

1. Stir or shake can of full-fat coconut milk to distribute contents evenly. Pour about ½ cup or so of the can (you don't have to be exact) into saucepan. Add canned salmon to saucepan. Add sea salt, basil, and ginger. Add water to get desired soup consistency and heat. When soup is heated, add coconut oil.

Tips

For a spicier dish add chili pepper or curry powder.

163. Tomato Soup

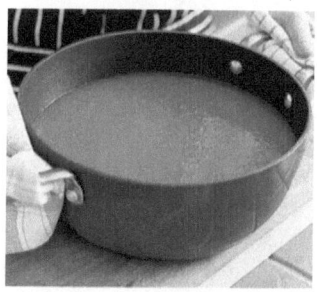

Stevia is a great sugar substitute. It is a good digestive aid and in more than 500 scientific studies, has shown no negative effects.

Ingredients

- 1 8 oz. can tomato sauce
- ½ cup chicken broth
- 3 tbsp. heavy cream

- 1 tsp sea salt
- ½ tsp pepper
- 1 tsp stevia sweetener
- ¼ cup cheese, grated

Method

1. Pour tomato sauce into small saucepan. Add chicken broth and heavy cream. Add stevia, sea salt, and black pepper to taste. Heat through and top with grated cheese.

Notes

This soup is ready quickly and nice on a chilly winter's day. You can enjoy it, knowing you won't be ingesting all the needless carbs and sugar that regular canned Cream of Tomato Soup contains.

But it tastes just as delicious and is chock full of lycopene from the cooked tomatoes, a potent anti-cancer weapon.

164. Coconut Crusted Salmon

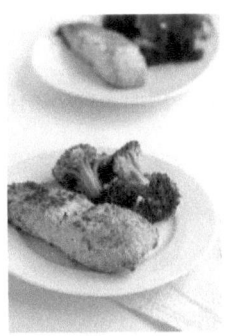

Eating salmon is important due to the depletion of minerals from our soil. Salmon provides an abundance of vitamins A and D and trace minerals such as iodine and zinc.

Ingredients

- Salmon filets
- 2 eggs, beaten
- 1 cup dried coconut
- 1 tsp sea salt
- 1 tsp garlic powder

- 1 tsp parsley flakes
- ½ tsp cayenne pepper
- 1 tsp onion powder
- Salt and pepper

Method

1. Dip fresh or thawed salmon fillets into beaten eggs. Place coconut flakes, salt and pepper, parsley flakes, onion powder, garlic powder, and cayenne pepper in a blender. Blend until fine and pour breading mix onto large dinner plate. Coat chicken pieces generously with faux breading by laying each side of salmon in the crumbs. Grease baking dish and lay filets singularly on dish. Bake at 350 until meat is tender and breading is crispy, approximately 30 minutes.

Notes

There is no need to worry about mercury when you eat deep sea fish like Alaskan Salmon.

165. Peanut Crusted Chicken

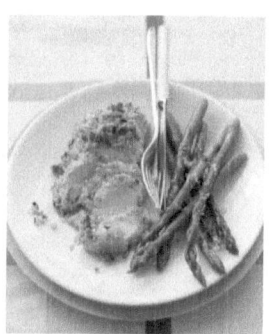

This recipe works fantastically with boneless chicken thigh tenderloins, but breast tenderloins are fine also.

Ingredients

- 6 boneless chicken breasts or thighs
- 1 cup sugar-free peanut butter
- ¼ cup water
- 2 tbsp. coconut oil
- ½ tsp salt

- 1 tsp black pepper
- ¼ red pepper flakes
- ½ tsp onion powder

Method

1. Pre-cook chicken boneless breasts or thighs by poaching in a pot with water, or bake in a covered tray until nearly tender. In a small bowl, mix peanut butter with water using a whisk. Add coconut oil, red pepper, salt, black pepper, and onion powder. Mix all sauce ingredients together.

2. Place cooked chicken pieces on large dinner plate and pour peanut sauce on top. Using your hands, toss chicken around in the sauce, making sure all pieces are well covered. Messy, but fun. Place coated chicken on greased baking sheet. Broil on middle rack, turning chicken a couple of times so both sides become nicely browned and very crispy.

Notes

An alternative way to make this recipe is to use uncooked chicken breast tenderloins, coat them in the sauce, and fry them in coconut oil. They still taste delicious, but it takes longer for those with large families, as you'll have to do multiple batches.

166. Cheeseburger Pie

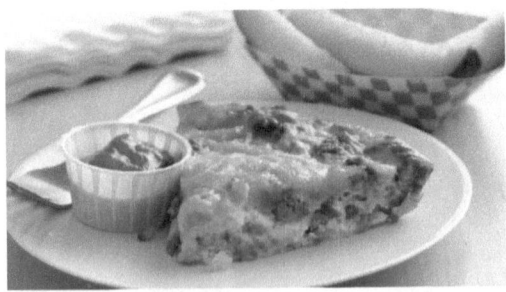

There are many versions of this basic recipe floating around. That's because we all have our own ideas of what a perfect cheeseburger should be like. Basically, anyway you like your cheeseburger can apply to this pie. You could include a layer of finely diced sautéed onions, dill pickles, jalapeños, or even a layer of tomatoes.

Ingredients

- 2 pounds ground beef
- 1 tsp salt
- 3 tsp onion powder
- 12 oz. grated cheese
- 2 eggs
- ½ cup mayonnaise
- ½ cup heavy cream
- ½ cup onions, chopped
- ½ tsp pepper

Method

1. Brown 2 lbs. beef and drain fat. Add onion powder and salt. Place beef mixture in casserole dish and stir in 6 oz. grated cheese. Place layer of any optional ingredients over beef and cheese combination, or skip this step for a more basic pie. In another bowl beat eggs, mayo, heavy cream, salt, and pepper. Pour mix over beef and top with another 6-oz. cheese. Bake at 350 for 35 minutes.

Notes

Serve with either, or both, a side salad and steamed buttery vegetables. Alternatively, use 1 packet onion soup mix instead of onion powder and salt for a fantastic taste.

167. Broccoli Cheese Soup

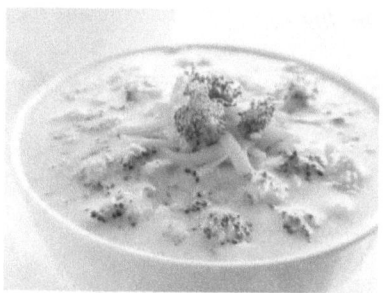

This soup can be the makings of a full evening meal if your family is smaller. If you have a larger family, double the recipe and throw in a little diced cooked chicken breast at the end to increase the protein content, or use some from a can.

Ingredients

- ½ cup water
- 4 cups chicken broth
- 8 oz. cream cheese
- 1/3 cup heavy cream
- ½ tsp salt
- ½ tsp cayenne pepper
- 6 oz. grated chees
- 2 frozen (12 oz.) packages of broccoli, or two heads of fresh broccoli, steamed

Method

1. Put steamed broccoli into blender in batches with just enough water to enable it to blend smoothly. You may keep some broccoli aside if you want some chunkiness to the soup. Pour blended broccoli into a pot with chicken broth. Add cream cheese and heavy cream. Season generously with salt, pepper, and cayenne pepper. Add more water to create a soupy consistency. Simmer for 5 minutes. Top with grated cheese.

Notes

This blending idea can turn any non-starchy vegetable into a creamy soup. Cauliflower and squash also work well. It's even more amazing if you pre-bake them with butter rather than steam before blending.

If you don't want to use cream cheese, use more chicken broth and add regular grated cheese into the soup.

168. Chicken Broccoli Casserole

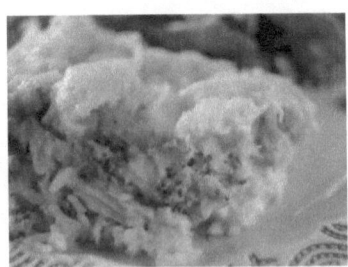

Some people hate eating broccoli on its own, but they like a cheesy casserole.

Ingredients

- 2 cups water or chicken broth
- 1 cup uncooked rice
- 4 chicken breasts, cooked and diced
- 8 oz. cheese, shredded
- 1 head fresh broccoli, florets only
- 1 tsp salt
- 1 tsp pepper
- 1 tsp garlic powder

Method

1. Place uncooked rice in casserole dish and cover with water. Add chicken, broccoli, and spices. Top with cheese. Bake, covered, at 350 degrees for 45 minutes.

Notes

Not only is this dish healthy for you as it is filled with greens and vitamins, but including broccoli, or other cruciferous veggies like cauliflower, brussels sprouts, and cabbage in several meals each week has been shown to reduce breast cancer risk.

169. Cheesecake

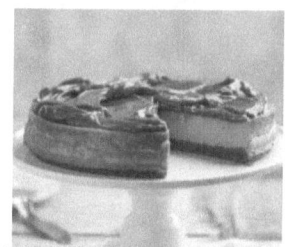

This basic recipe is crust-less. You will probably not miss the crust, but if you do, simply throw some finely chopped nuts or ground almond meal on the baking dish before pouring in the cheesecake mixture.

Ingredients

- 2 8 oz. packages cream cheese
- 2 eggs
- ½ cup stevia sweetener

- ½ tsp vanilla extract
- Juice from ½ lemon or 1 T lemon juice concentrate

Method

1. Place cream cheese into mixing bowl. Add 2 eggs, stevia, vanilla, and lemon juice. Beat well with electric beater for 3-5 minutes. Pour mix into small greased baking dish.

2. Place this dish in a bigger roasting pan with some water that comes up halfway on your cheesecake pan (the water surrounds the outside of the dish in which you are baking your cheesecake). This is a water bath and will stop your cheesecake from sinking in the middle. Bake at 350 for approximately 30 minutes.

Notes

Berries can be added to the cheesecake if you desire. You can also make mini cheesecakes from this mixture by putting the mix in well-greased muffin pans.

The mini cheesecakes do sink in the middle, but that becomes a perfect space for adding the berries.

170. Peanut Squares

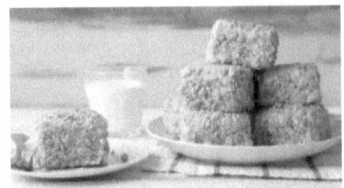

Delicious!

Ingredients

- 1 cup almond flour
- ½ cup dry roasted peanuts, finely chopped
- ¼ cup butter, melted
- ½ cup stevia sweetener
- 12 oz. cream cheese
- 2/3 cup peanut butter
- ¾ cup heavy cream

Method

1. Put 1 cup almond flour in bowl. Add dry roasted peanuts, butter, and ½ stevia sweetener. Mix together well. Press mixed ingredients into greased 8-inch baking dish and bake for 10-15 minutes at 350F. While crust is baking, put cream cheese and the remaining stevia sweetener into a bowl and beat until light and fluffy. Add peanut butter and beat some more.

2. In separate bowl, beat heavy cream and fold into the cream cheese mixture. Top cooled crust with mixture and place dessert in refrigerator to chill.

171. Chocolate Cupcakes

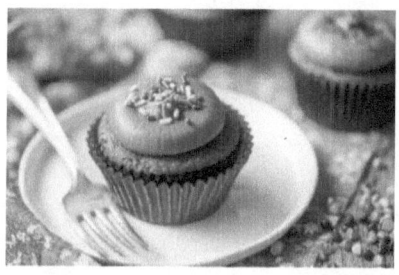

This recipe makes six muffins. You can use Greek yogurt in place of sour cream if you prefer.

Ingredients

- 3 eggs
- ¼ cup unsweetened cocoa powder
- 2 tsp baking powder
- 1 cup stevia sweetener
- 3 tbsp. water
- 1/8 cup sour cream
- 3 tbsp. coconut oil, melted

Method

1. Crack eggs into a bowl and whisk. Add cocoa powder and baking powder. Add water and sour cream, coconut oil, and stevia sweetener. Whisk ingredients well and pour into greased muffin tin. Bake for 12-15 minutes at 350 or until tops are just done.

Notes

These are a great dessert to serve to visitors. Adorn with cut strawberries and whipped cream. Very impressive!

172. Blueberry Coffee Cake

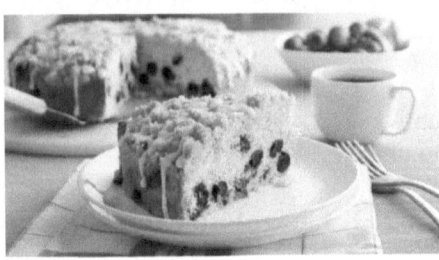

This cake isn't just for breakfast, but is delicious any time of day.

Ingredients

- 3 eggs, beaten
- 3 cups fresh or frozen blueberries
- ½ cup milk
- 1 cup stevia sweetener
- 1 ½ cups almond flour
- 2 tbsp. coconut oil, melted
- 1 tsp vanilla extract
- ½ tsp salt
- ½ tsp nutmeg
- 1 tbsp. cinnamon
- 1 tsp baking soda

Method

1. Mix dry ingredients. Mix eggs, milk, coconut oil, and vanilla extract. Add to dry ingredients and mix well. Fold in the blueberries. Place mixture in greased 8-inch baking dish and bake at 350 degrees for 25 minutes.

Notes

You could substitute two mashed bananas for the blueberries in this recipe and add ½ cup chopped walnuts.

Conclusion

You don't have time, but this should not be the reason why you want to prepare and eat unhealthy meals. As far as eating low calorie healthy foods is concerned, it can be a hassle finding the right foods, but it really helps if you know what to look for. Most importantly, each and every low-calorie recipe in this book is fast, low cost and less than 300 calories per serving.

For weight loss control, the best bet is healthy meals that provide low energy with high volume. The recipes in this book are high in volume so that you can eat more and feel fuller on fewer calories all day long. If you are truly watching your weight then you definitely want to make sensible choices with our low-calorie recipes.

Final Words

I would like to thank you for downloading my book and I hope I have been able to help you and educate you about something new.

If you have enjoyed this book and would like to share your positive thoughts, could you please take 30 seconds of your time to go back and give me a review on my Amazon book page!

I greatly appreciate seeing these reviews because it helps me share my hard work!

Again, thank you and I wish you all the best with your cooking journey!

Last Chance to Get YOUR Bonus!

FOR A LIMITED TIME ONLY – Get Olivia's best-selling book *"The #1 Cookbook: Over 170+ of the Most Popular Recipes Across 7 Different Cuisines!"* absolutely FREE!

Readers have absolutely loved this book because of the wide variety of recipes. It is highly recommended you check these recipes out and see what you can add to your home menu!

Once again, as a big thank-you for downloading this book, I'd like to offer it to you *100% FREE for a LIMITED TIME ONLY!*

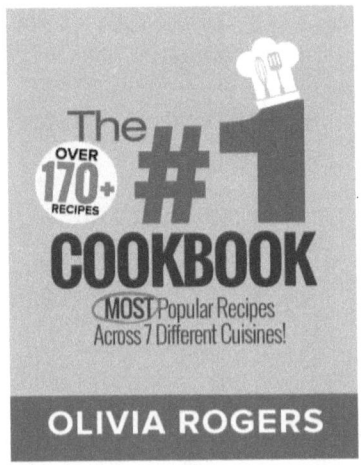

Get your free copy at:

TheMenuAtHome.com/Bonus

Disclaimer

This book and related site provides recipe and food advice in an informative and educational manner only, with information that is general in nature and that is not specific to you, the reader. The contents of this book and related site are intended to assist you and other readers in your personal efforts. Consult your physician or nutritionist regarding the applicability of any information provided in our information to you.

Nothing in this book should be construed as personal advice or diagnosis, and must not be used in this manner. The information provided about conditions is general in nature. This information does not cover all possible uses, actions, precautions, side-effects, or interactions of medicines, or medical procedures. The information in this site should not be considered as complete and does not cover all diseases, ailments, physical conditions, or their treatment.

No Warranties: The authors and publishers don't guarantee or warrant the quality, accuracy, completeness, timeliness, appropriateness or suitability of the information in this book, or of any product or services referenced by this site.

The information in this site is provided on an "as is" basis and the authors and publishers make no representations or warranties of any kind with respect to this information. This site may contain inaccuracies, typographical errors, or other errors.

Liability Disclaimer: The publishers, authors, and other parties involved in the creation, production, provision of information, or delivery of this site specifically disclaim any responsibility, and shall not be held liable for any damages, claims, injuries, losses, liabilities, costs, or obligations including any direct, indirect, special, incidental, or consequences damages (collectively known as "Damages") whatsoever and howsoever caused, arising out of, or in connection with the use or misuse of the site and the information contained within it, whether such Damages arise in contract, tort, negligence, equity, statute law, or by way of other legal theory.

www.ingramcontent.com/pod-product-compliance
Lightning Source LLC
Chambersburg PA
CBHW031110080526
44587CB00011B/911